Outcomes Measures in Plastic Surgery

Editors

KEVIN C. CHUNG
ANDREA L. PUSIC

CLINICS IN PLASTIC SURGERY

www.plasticsurgery.theclinics.com

April 2013 • Volume 40 • Number 2

ELSEVIER

1600 John F. Kennedy Boulevard • Suite 1800 • Philadelphia, Pennsylvania, 19103-2899

http://www.theclinics.com

CLINICS IN PLASTIC SURGERY Volume 40, Number 2
April 2013 ISSN 0094-1298, ISBN-13: 978-1-4557-7141-7

Editor: Joanne Husovski
Development Editor: Donald Mumford

Clinics in Plastic Surgery (ISSN 0094-1298) is published quarterly by Elsevier Inc., 360 Park Avenue South, New York, NY 10010-1710. Months of issue are January, April, July, and October. Business and Editorial Offices: 1600 John F. Kennedy Blvd., Suite 1800, Philadelphia, PA 19103-2899. Periodicals postage paid at New York, NY and additional mailing offices. Subscription prices are $466.00 per year for US individuals, $693.00 per year for US institutions, $229.00 per year for US students and residents, $529.00 per year for Canadian individuals, $809.00 per year for Canadian institutions, $607.00 per year for international individuals, $809.00 per year for international institutions, and $289.00 per year for Canadian and foreign students/residents. To receive student/resident rate, orders must be accompanied by name of affiliated institution, date of term, and the *signature* of program/residency coordinator on institution letterhead. Orders will be billed at individual rate until proof of status is received. Foreign air speed delivery is included in all *Clinics* subscription prices. All prices are subject to change without notice. **POSTMASTER:** Send address changes to *Clinics in Plastic Surgery*, Elsevier Health Sciences Division, Subscription Customer Service, 3251 Riverport Lane, Maryland Heights, MO 63043. **Customer Service: 1-800-654-2452 (US and Canada). From outside of the United States and Canada, call 314-447-8871. Fax: 314-447-8029. E-mail: JournalsCustomerService-usa@elsevier.com (for print support); JournalsOnlineSupport-usa@elsevier.com (for online support).**

Reprints. For copies of 100 or more of articles in this publication, please contact the Commercial Reprints Department, Elsevier Inc., 360 Park Avenue South, New York, New York 10010-1710. Tel.: (+1) 212-633-3812; Fax: (+1) 212-462-1935; E-mail: reprints@elsevier.com.

Clinics in Plastic Surgery is covered in *Current Contents, EMBASE/Excerpta Medica, Science Citation Index, MEDLINE/ PubMed (Index Medicus), ASCA,* and *ISI/BIOMED.*

Printed and bound by CPI Group (UK) Ltd, Croydon, CR0 4YY
Transferred to Digital Printing, 2013

Contributors

EDITORS

KEVIN C. CHUNG, MD, MS
Professor of Surgery, Assistant Dean for
Faculty Affairs, Section of Plastic Surgery,
Department of Surgery, University of Michigan,
The University of Michigan Health System,
Ann Arbor, Michigan

ANDREA L. PUSIC, MD, MHS, FRCSC, FACS
Associate Professor, Plastic and
Reconstructive Surgical Service, Memorial
Sloan-Kettering Cancer Center, New York,
New York

AUTHORS

CLAUDIA R. ALBORNOZ, MD, MSc
Plastic and Reconstructive Surgical Service,
Memorial Sloan-Kettering Cancer Center,
New York, New York

AMY ALDERMAN, MD, MPH, FACS
Private Practice, Atlanta, Georgia

STEFAN J. CANO, PhD
Clinical Neurology Research Group, Plymouth
University Peninsula Schools of Medicine and
Dentistry, Plymouth, United Kingdom

KEVIN C. CHUNG, MD, MS
Professor of Surgery, Assistant Dean for
Faculty Affairs, Section of Plastic Surgery,
Department of Surgery, University of Michigan,
The University of Michigan Health System,
Ann Arbor, Michigan

PETER G. CORDEIRO, MD
Plastic and Reconstructive Surgical Service,
Memorial Sloan-Kettering Cancer Center,
New York, New York

**CHRISTOPHER R. FORREST, MD, MSc,
FRCSC**
Chief, Interim Chair and Professor, Division of
Plastic and Reconstructive Surgery,
Department of Surgery, Medical Director,
HSC Centre for Craniofacial Care and
Research, Hospital for Sick Children,
Faculty of Medicine, University of Toronto,
Toronto, Ontario, Canada

AVIRAM M. GILADI, MD
Resident, Section of Plastic Surgery,
Department of Surgery, The University of
Michigan Health System, Ann Arbor,
Michigan

TIM E.E. GOODACRE, MBBS, BSc, FRCS
Honorary Senior Lecturer, Clinical Medicine,
Consultant Plastic Surgeon, The Spires
Cleft Centre, Oxford Radcliffe Children's
Hospital, University of Oxford, Headley Way;
Chair, BAPRAS Professional Standards
Committee, Headington, Oxford,
United Kingdom

ANNE F. KLASSEN, DPhil, BA
Faculty of Health Sciences, Associate
Professor and Member, Department of
Pediatrics, Clinical Epidemiology &
Biostatistics, McMaster University, Hamilton,
Ontario, Canada

EVAN KOWALSKI, BS
Section of Plastic Surgery,
Department of Surgery, The University of
Michigan Health System, Ann Arbor,
Michigan

VALERIE LEMAINE, MD, MPH, FRCSC
Assistant Professor, Division of Plastic
Surgery, Department of Surgery, Mayo Clinic,
Rochester, Minnesota

SUNITHA MALAY, MPH
Clinical Research Coordinator, Section of
Plastic Surgery, Department of Surgery,
The University of Michigan Health System,
Ann Arbor, Michigan

EVAN MATROS, MD, MMSc
Plastic and Reconstructive Surgical Service,
Memorial Sloan-Kettering Cancer Center,
New York, New York

COLLEEN MCCARTHY, MD, MS, FRCSC
Assistant Attending Surgeon, Department of
Surgery, Memorial Sloan-Kettering Cancer
Center, New York, New York

ADEYIZA O. MOMOH, MD
Clinical Assistant Professor, Section of Plastic
Surgery, The University of Michigan Health
System, Ann Arbor, Michigan

ANDREA L. PUSIC, MD, MHS, FRCSC, FACS
Associate Professor, Plastic and
Reconstructive Surgical Service, Memorial
Sloan-Kettering Cancer Center, New York,
New York

PATRICK REAVEY, MD
Plastic and Reconstructive Surgical Service,
Memorial Sloan-Kettering Cancer Center,
New York, New York

AMIE M. SCOTT, MPH
Plastic and Reconstructive Surgical Service,
Memorial Sloan-Kettering Cancer Center,
New York, New York

MELISSA J. SHAUVER, MPH
Clinical Research Coordinator, Section of
Plastic Surgery, Department of Surgery,
The University of Michigan Health System,
Ann Arbor, Michigan

JENNIFER F. WALJEE, MD, MS
Assistant Professor, Section of Plastic Surgery,
Department of Surgery, The University of
Michigan Health System, Ann Arbor,
Michigan

KAREN W.Y. WONG, MD, MSc, FRCSC
Clinical and Research Fellow in Pediatric
Plastic Surgery, Division of Plastic Surgery,
Department of Surgery, Hospital for Sick
Children, University of Toronto, Toronto,
Ontario, Canada

TONI ZHONG, MD, MHS, FRCSC
Assistant Professor, Division of Plastic and
Reconstructive Surgery, Department of
Surgery and Surgical Oncology,
University of Toronto, Toronto, Ontario,
Canada

Contents

Evidence-based medicine is analyzed from its inception. This article takes the reader through the early formation of scientific medicine that has evolved into the multipurpose tool it has become today. Early proponents of evidence-based medicine and the outcomes movement, and their intentions, are presented. The work of David Sackett, Gordon Guyatt, Florence Nightingale, Ernest Codman, and Archie Cochrane is discussed, regarding how they perceived the need for better clinical outcomes that led to a more formalized evidence-based practice. The fundamentals are discussed objectively in detail, and potential flaws are presented that guide the reader to deeper comprehension.

Satisfaction with appearance and improved quality of life are key outcomes for patients undergoing facial aesthetic procedures. The FACE-Q is a new patient-reported outcome (PRO) instrument encompassing a suite of independently functioning scales designed to measure a range of important outcomes for facial aesthetics patients. FACE-Q scales were developed with strict adherence to international guidelines for PRO instrument development. This article describes the development and psychometric evaluation of the core FACE-Q scale, the Satisfaction with Facial Appearance scale. Both modern and traditional psychometric methods were used to confirm that this new 10-item scale is a reliable, valid, and responsive measure.

Patient-reported outcomes serve as an essential and perhaps more relevant means for assessing patients' response to treatment than clinical measures alone. Many of the procedures performed in plastic surgery are associated with aesthetic outcomes. Therefore, it is pertinent to thoroughly understand the patient's perspective of achieved results. Surgeons need to possess knowledge and skills about outcomes assessments and understand how to apply them to improve quality of care delivered based on evidence. This article discusses the appropriate use of outcome questionnaires to rigorously evaluate treatment methods based on patient satisfaction and the outcome measurement instruments frequently used in plastic surgery.

In recent decades, the expansion of health services research has created an opportunity to crate salient, evidence-based guidelines for diagnosis, treatment, and prognosis. However, for many aspects of care, incorporation of new scientific knowledge into clinical practice often lags, particularly among the surgical subspecialties. This article highlights the development of evidence-based medicine, the principles of innovation diffusion, and successes and challenges in developing plastic surgery quality initiatives.

This article presents an introduction to economic outcomes for the plastic surgeon investigator. Types of economic outcomes are introduced and the matter of perspective is discussed. Examples from the plastic surgery literature are presented. The current and future importance of economic outcome measures is emphasized.

The BREAST-Q© is a multiscale, multimodule, patient-reported outcome instrument (PRO) measuring health-related quality of life and patient satisfaction in women who undergo breast surgery. This PRO instrument is the flagship of our team's research, which has spanned almost a decade. This article provides detail about the BREAST-Q©. The BREAST-Q© represents a significant advance in measuring the impact and effectiveness of breast surgery from the patients' perspective. In addition, our overall approach may provide a useful template for the development of future PRO instruments.

The article presents an objective view of evidence-based medicine application to aesthetic surgery. The challenges are discussed and the points that create them are analyzed. Psychological and external factors in decision-making for aesthetic surgery are presented. The handling of surgical complications is presented as an example affecting reporting of outcomes.

This article discusses the measurement of outcomes in craniofacial and pediatric plastic surgery, using examples of craniosynostosis and cleft lip and/or palate (CLP). The challenges in measuring the standard outcomes of function, aesthetics, and health-related quality of life are discussed, along with the importance of developing evidence and studying quality improvement in this specialty. The need to define specific and comprehensive goals is discussed with a focus on patient-reported outcomes (PROs). Examples from the development of the CLEFT-Q, a PRO instrument for patients with CLP, are provided to support the need to seek the patient perspective.

CLINICS IN PLASTIC SURGERY

Erratum

In the article, Preoperative Evaluation of the Brow-Lid Continuum by Craig N. Czyz, DO, Robert H. Hill, MD, and Jill A. Foster, MD in the January 2013 issue by Azizzadeh and Massry, the red line in Figure 1B is intended to state "MRD$_1$."

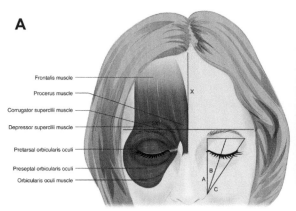

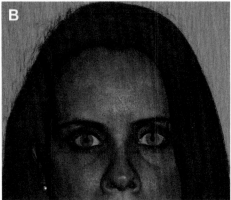

Fig. 1. (A) Facial musculature pertinent to the brow-lid continuum. Markings on the forehead indicate what some consider the "ideal" brow contour. The forehead should be 2× in horizontal length as vertical height (×). The lines drawn from the nasal ala through the periocular landmarks to the brow represent the idea position of (A) brow origin (medial canthus); (B) maximal arch (lateral limbus); (C). Brow tail termination (lateral canthus). (B) Vertical height of eyebrows. Black = VPF; Red = MRD$_1$; Purple = MBD.

http://dx.doi.org/10.1016/j.cps.2013.01.001
0094-1298/13/$ – see front matter

plasticsurgery.theclinics.com

Erratum

In the article, Preoperative Evaluation of the ... the January 2013 issue by Alizadeh and Broumand Continuum by Craig N. Czyz, DO, ... Massry, the red line in Figure 18 is intended to ... Robert H. Hill, MD, and Jill A. Foster, MD in ... state "MRD".

Fig. 1. (a) Facial musculature pertinent to the brow-lid continuum. Markings on the forehead indicate what some consider the "ideal" brow contour. The forehead should be 2x in horizontal length as vertical height. (x) The lines drawn from the nasal ala through the periocular landmarks to the brow represent the idea position of (2A) brow origin (medial canthus), (B) maximal arch (lateral limbus), (C) & low tail termination (lateral canthus). (B) Vertical height of eyebrows. Black = VPF, Red = MRD, Purple = MRD ...

Preface
Patient-Reported Outcomes Instruments

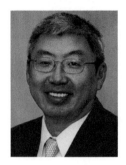 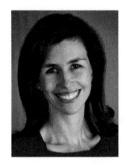

Kevin C. Chung, MD, MS   Andrea L. Pusic, MD, MHS, FRCSC
Editors

It is truly an honor for us to serve as editors of this volume on Outcomes for Surgical Guidance in Plastic Surgery. As developers of patient-reported outcomes (PRO) instruments, we have a special interest in this area and have been pleased to see the increasing quantity and quality of patient-centric research in plastic surgery.

The Michigan Hand Outcome Questionnaire (MHQ) was developed when the use of PRO instruments was still in its infancy; however, after many years of clinical application, the MHQ has become a standard by which outcomes in hand surgery are judged. As we move forward, important advancements are being made in the ways that PRO instruments are developed. Specifically, there is strong emphasis on developing scales that can provide clinically meaningful data and effectively measure change. Condition-specific outcome instruments, such as the Breast-Q and Face-Q, have recently been developed using in-depth qualitative research and new psychometric methods such as Rasch. These "next generation" PRO instruments offer the potential to rigorously quantify outcomes from our patients' perspective to inform technical advancement and clinical care. In fact, new PRO instruments are so responsive to clinical change that government agencies such as the National Institutes of Health and the Food and Drug Administration are investing substantial resources to apply their use to measure the effectiveness of current and new treatments. Internationally, many countries are now starting to require that new devices and medications present PRO data before new medical products are approved.

Because Plastic Surgery is a specialty that addresses quality of life issues for patients with a variety of diseases and conditions, the application of PRO instruments is particularly pertinent to measure functional as well as psychosocial changes after treatment. In this volume, we have invited some of the top scientists in outcomes research to share with you the current status of outcomes instrument design and selection in all disciplines of Plastic Surgery. These articles were written not in a dry, pedantic academic fashion, but in a relevant manner so that the readers can apply these principles in their daily practices to assess outcomes in their patients. For researchers interested in outcomes research, these articles are necessary reading when embarking on a critical assessment of outcomes of a particular device or treatment.

We trust that as the outcomes movement continues to evolve, there will be ever more innovative studies using new PRO instruments to better delineate and understand patients' perceptions of the treatments they receive. This will be accomplished in part by leveraging electronic and web-based data capture. In addition, we now seek to

Clin Plastic Surg 40 (2013) xi–xii
http://dx.doi.org/10.1016/j.cps.2012.10.010
0094-1298/13/$ – see front matter

plasticsurgery.theclinics.com

measure not only quality of life, but also our patients' expectations and satisfaction. As Plastic Surgery continues to embrace outcomes research and evidence-based medicine, we hope that our field will take a leading role in designing and applying PRO instruments. After all, Plastic Surgery is a quality-of-life specialty, and its mission is to enhance patients' well-being through a careful consideration of the functional, aesthetic, and psychosocial welfare of the patients we treat.

Kevin C. Chung, MD, MS
University of Michigan
Ann Arbor, MI, USA

Andrea L. Pusic, MD, MHS, FRCSC
Memorial Sloan Kettering Hospital
New York, NY, USA

E-mail addresses:
kecchung@med.umich.edu (K.C. Chung)
PusicA@mskcc.org (A.L. Pusic)

The Outcomes Movement and Evidence-Based Medicine in Plastic Surgery

Evan Kowalski, BS[a], Kevin C. Chung, MD, MS[b],*

KEYWORDS

• Evidence-based medicine • Outcomes • Historical review • Principles and flaws • Plastic surgery

KEY POINTS

- At its core, evidence-based medicine attempts to bridge the gap between the realms of research and practice.
- A recent poll in the *British Medical Journal* selected evidence-based medicine as 1 of the 15 greatest milestones in medicine since 1840, alongside medical advances such as antibiotics and vaccines.
- Despite its nearly universal acceptance and approval by numerous authorities, clinicians and academicians must remain diligent to prevent the abuse of evidence-based medicine.
- Although the outcomes movement has gathered considerable momentum in the medical research sector, its application has not halted the continued escalation of health care costs and the uncertain quality of medical services.
- Physicians are increasingly aware that the randomized controlled trial is not the only form of valid study, and it is becoming clear that these studies must be performed in conjunction with observational studies to find the best evidence.

OVERVIEW

While counseling his students more than 2500 years ago, Hippocrates declared that the physician need to "rely on actual evidence rather than on conclusions resulting solely from reasoning, because arguments in the form of idle words are erroneous and can be easily refuted."[1] Since the early days of medicine, there has been a need for evidence-based inquiries that enable a physician to ascertain and apply the best treatment strategy for each patient. Even during the early era of medicine, physicians understood the importance of using evidence to guide treatment protocols. Although we identify the outcomes movement and evidence-based medicine as new terms, the ideas that embody these themes are as old as organized medicine itself. Increased government involvement combined with an exceedingly demanding patient population have made the modern outcomes movement and evidence-based medicine an essential component of research and clinical practice.

Supported in part by grants from the National Institute on Aging and National Institute of Arthritis and Musculoskeletal and Skin Diseases (R01 AR062066), and from the National Institute of Arthritis and Musculoskeletal and Skin Diseases (2R01 AR047328-06) and a Midcareer Investigator Award in Patient-Oriented Research (K24 AR053120) (to Dr Kevin C. Chung).
[a] Section of Plastic Surgery, Department of Surgery, The University of Michigan Health System, 1500 East Medical Center Drive, Ann Arbor, MI 48109-5340, USA; [b] Section of Plastic Surgery, The University of Michigan Medical School, 2130 Taubman Center, SPC 5340, 1500 East Medical Center Drive, Ann Arbor, MI 48109-5340, USA
* Corresponding author.
E-mail address: kecchung@umich.edu

EARLY EVIDENCE-BASED MEDICINE MOVEMENT

The outcomes movement and evidence-based medicine were spurred on by many early proponents, some of whom were shunned by their peers in response to the radical new ideas that they imposed. During the 1800s, the celebrated nurse Florence Nightingale used evidence gained from careful record keeping, observation, and statistical measurements to foster health care reform, becoming one of the earliest supporters of evidence-based medicine.[2] Ernest Codman advocated meticulous data collection, patient follow-up, and the analysis and interpretation of patient outcomes to improve care and treatment methods. Although his ideas had practical value, his peers did not share his enthusiasm for the improvement of outcomes, instead preferring to alienate the brilliant surgeon and continue using the dated techniques and treatment methods they had learned during their medical training.[3,4] Archie Cochrane championed the use of rigorously performed randomized controlled trials (RCTs) and systematic reviews, sparking the interest of those who would go on to place them at the top of the research hierarchy.[5] Although they did not articulate these efforts in a particular terminology, these early pioneers were instrumental in the implementation of outcomes research and evidence-based methodology in medicine.

MODERN EVIDENCE-BASED MEDICINE MOVEMENT

The modern outcomes movement in the United States has its roots in the Era of Expansion of the 1950s and 1960s, which stimulated a massive overhaul of the medical industry. This period was distinguished by a substantial increase in the number of medical facilities and physicians, extraordinary advances in science and medical technology, and for the first time an augmentation of medical insurance coverage into the majority of United States households. These changes created a different hospital system, attracting private investors who were looking to increase profit margins. The increased demand for medical services coupled with the high expenses incurred from sophisticated medical technology led to a substantial increase in medical costs. The soaring cost of medical care caused a crisis whereby patients began to demand lower prices for medical services. Also feeling the burden of high costs, the federal government and employers followed suit and started dictating the costs of health care, paying the hospitals much less than they were charging for the services that were being provided.

At the same time, the American public began to question the quality of the new, high-tech, and expensive treatment protocols that were quickly becoming standard practice. The Era of Expansion initially generated a belief that by increasing hospital admittance rates the overall population would be healthier, a belief that was later found invalid. Several investigators documented the variations in health care among different regions and hospitals, and soon established that high admittance rates and medical costs do not always translate to better medical care and a healthier population.[6–11] These studies also raised concerns over the impact these substantial variations in health care might have on a population.[12–16] Areas with easy access to health care and high admittance rates may have increased rates of unnecessary procedures, resulting in higher rates of preventable complications and increased medical costs. Populations in areas with low admittance rates may experience difficulty obtaining access to care and may not benefit from the advances of modern medicine. Because of the high variability of medical and surgical services among practitioners, hospitals, and regions, the optimal rate of hospital admittance and surgical interventions for different patients and conditions remains to be determined. This research avenue demands continued exploration so that costs can be contained and health care among all populations simultaneously improved.

MOMENTUM OF EVIDENCE-BASED STRATEGIES IN THE MEDICAL COMMUNITY

Although the outcomes movement has gathered considerable momentum in the medical research sector, its application has not halted the continued escalation of health care costs and the uncertain quality of medical services. Even so, the outcomes movement has played an important role in paving the way for the widespread implementation and acceptance of evidence-based strategies into the medical community. In fact, evidence-based medicine was specifically designed to address the shortcomings that are apparent in the outcomes movement by focusing simply on the application of outcomes data rather than on the scientific rigor of deriving these outcomes data. Physicians David Sackett and Gordon Guyatt would lay the initial groundwork for the development of evidence-based medicine, and both would go on to provide substantial contributions to the continued evolution of the concept.

While studying ways to improve treatment compliance of hypertension in 1975, Sackett discovered a disturbing trend. He and the other investigators found that a determining factor in the prescribing treatment for hypertension was the graduating year of the physician. It appeared that the treating physicians were basing their management of patients on the treatment protocol that was considered acceptable at the time they had completed their medical training, even if the treatment was completely outdated.[17] This recurring theme prompted David Sackett, Brian Haynes, Peter Tugwell, and Victor Neufeld to publish a series of articles beginning in 1981 in the *Canadian Medical Association Journal* highlighting the importance of a physician's ability to carefully read and comprehend research published in medical journals.[18] In this series of articles, the investigators emphasize using epidemiology concepts to apply the best available evidence and solve clinical problems. These articles were aimed at helping the busy clinician stay up to date with the latest advances in medicine.

The phrase "evidence-based medicine" was initially coined in 1990 by Gordon Guyatt, after an unsuccessful attempt to implement a new strategy he originally defined "Scientific Medicine" into an internal medicine residency program at McMasters University. His Scientific Medicine program was designed to enhance clinical treatment with the application of current systematic scientific evidence, modeled after the ideas of his mentor David Sackett. The program was promptly disparaged by his peers, who were offended at the implication that current decision-making practices in medicine lacked scientific qualities.[19] This reaction persuaded Guyatt to give his initiative a new designation: evidence-based medicine. With this new name his proposed residency program curriculum was well received, compelling Guyatt to officially publish the term in a 1991 editorial.[20] Not long after, a team at McMasters University, including Sackett and Guyatt, continued improving on the idea of evidence-based medicine, eventually leading to an international collaboration between Canadian and American academicians to further enhance this novel approach.

INTERNATIONAL EVIDENCE-BASED MEDICINE WORKING GROUP

The International Evidence-Based Medicine Working Group, as it became known, worked to further refine evidence-based medicine from Sackett's original critical appraisal articles and Guyatt's previous concepts. The Group discovered that although the critical appraisal articles were helpful in guiding clinicians to better understand the quality of evidence in scientific articles, they lacked instruction on applying the evidence

gained from scientific studies to the clinical setting. After addressing potential problems and enhancing the existing components of evidence-based medicine, an improved version was officially introduced in 1992, promoting the critical appraisal, identification, and application of scientific evidence.[21] This article was followed by the *JAMA User's Guide to the Medical Literature*, a publication initially designed to help physicians better understand the basic concepts of evidence-based medicine, later progressing to a series of 25 articles as the initiative evolved and gained acceptance.

EVIDENCE-BASED MEDICINE BRIDGES THE GAP BETWEEN RESEARCH AND PRACTICE

At its core, evidence-based medicine attempts to bridge the gap between the realms of research and practice. Although seemingly simple, this ideal is exceedingly complicated, plagued by countless arguments concerning effectiveness, a lack of procedural and technical comprehension, a pervasive fear of abuse, and an overabundance of poorly performed studies that hamper the use and quality of data. To account for these challenges and address the opposition to evidence-based medicine, Sackett and colleagues[22] published a short explanation titled "Evidence based medicine: what it is and what it isn't," which highlights the implications and importance of such a system. These investigators also explain that a good clinician must rely on individual experience and expertise, and incorporate the best available evidence to achieve the best possible outcomes, but that neither of these elements is sufficient in and of itself to provide the best care. Clinical experience is vital, but can quickly become outdated without the support of a good scientific knowledge base, whereas evidence alone can result in the poor management of a patient when the data are not applied appropriately, based on specific patient characteristics and needs. Thus, it is essential that physicians use both clinical experience and the best available evidence to provide the best treatment, a concept that has now been established as a fundamental principle for evidence-based practices.

FUNDAMENTAL PRINCIPLES OF EVIDENCE-BASED MEDICINE

In its current state, the *User's Guide to the Medical Literature* highlights not only the appraisal and application of the best available evidence but also the importance of patient preferences and values in terms of evidence-based medicine (**Fig. 1**).[23]

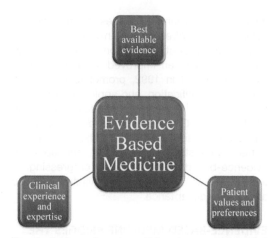

Fig. 1. Evidence-based medicine is comprised of 3 main components: the best available evidence, patient preferences and values, and clinical experience and expertise. These 3 elements must be used concurrently to successfully implement the concept of evidence-based medicine into clinical practice.

The second fundamental principle of evidence-based medicine is just as important as the first rule of collecting and analyzing evidence, and entails that "clinical decisions, recommendations, and practice guidelines must not only attend to the best available evidence, but also to the values and preferences of the informed patient."[24] Despite this property of evidence-based medicine and its overall prevalence, there is a gap between evidence-based medicine and preference-based medicine, and as more emphasis is put on patient-centered research and treatment, this gap must be narrowed to effectively satisfy the wants and needs of patients. In 2001, the Institute of Medicine asserted that patient-centered medical care based on the highest level of evidence is a critical aspect of high-quality health care.[25] It is far too often the case that clinicians and academicians forget or overlook this fundamental ideal of evidence-based medicine, but its importance cannot be overstated, especially for the patients who feel the direct effects of medical decisions.

One of the primary roles of the clinician is to provide each patient with essential background information about the patient's condition, including long-term effects with and without intervention, treatment options, and outcomes of therapeutic measures, in a way that is comprehensible to the patient. It is up to the physician to keep the patient and their family adequately informed so that he or she is capable of making a treatment decision that is most appropriate for the patient, based on the best available evidence as well as the patient's goals and values. It is not the job of a physician to push a specific treatment on the patient, but to

enable the patient to make an informed decision. As in evidence-based medicine, there are biases involved during decision making for the patient, and care must be taken to limit these influences. If the patient is optimistic about a treatment or potential involvement in a study, the physician must be careful to avoid selection bias by providing accurate information about the associated morbidity, risks, and complications of a particular regimen or procedure. A pessimistic patient must also be presented with accurate information about a treatment, but not in a way that would persuade the patient to accept the treatment. The physician must remember that, aside from emergency situations, he or she should only make recommendations, and it is the patient's decision of what treatment, if any, is to be used.

The paucity of RCTs in plastic surgery and the inability to perform some of these studies has left the field lacking level-1 evidence for many treatment options. It is apparent that this lack of evidence calls for an increase in the amount of research performed in plastic surgery but also that the evidence gained from this research must be appropriately applied to each individual patient's wants and needs. The surgical specialty has features that make it difficult to perform RCTs because a very specific set of expertise and systems is required to produce successful treatment results, but this does not mean it cannot be done. In the instance whereby a surgical treatment is eligible for investigation with an RCT, it is imperative that the treatment be standardized so as to prevent flawed results. For example, if a study were conducted on the different surgical treatment options available for distal radius fractures, each distinct surgical intervention would have to be performed in the same way by each participating surgeon. Plastic surgery has encountered a particularly difficult time in fully implementing the principles and practices that guide evidence-based medicine. One of the reasons why it is difficult to incorporate evidence-based medicine into plastic surgery is that it is not always possible to evaluate the outcomes of a profession that partially relies on artistic creativity. It is clear, however, that plastic surgeons can use evidence-based medicine in many ways, such as overcoming the excitement of using a novel surgical technique or new medical equipment before there are sufficient data to support its use.

FLAWS OF EVIDENCE-BASED MEDICINE

Evidence-based medicine is an invaluable asset in the pursuit of superior approaches to patient-centered care, but it has flaws. A common argument against evidence-based medicine is that it relies too heavily on the RCT as the best available evidence. Renowned physician and epidemiologist Alvan Feinstein argued that evidence-based medicine has the potential for major abuse, largely because the RCT is the foundation for the best available evidence. He stated that RCTs omit many clinical details that are essential in decision making, including "responses to previous therapeutic agents, short-term (24 hour) response to remedial therapy, ease of regulation when the dose must be 'titrated,' difficulty in compliance with therapy and reasons for noncompliance, psychic or nonclinical reasons for impaired functional status, the 'social support' system available at home and elsewhere, the patient's expectations and desires for therapeutic accomplishment, and the patient's psychological state and preferences."[26] In addition, he commented that a meta-analysis may be flawed if it is based on RCTs that are of low quality. This theme is not a new one, as even the early proponents of the meta-analysis have voiced their concern over the substantial effect the variable quality of RCTs can have on a pooled set of data.[27] Feinstein goes on to say that the studies demonstrating the effectiveness of penicillin and insulin were discovered in single study articles, and by the current standards of evidence-based medicine would be overlooked if reported today because of their low level on the research hierarchy. A poor-quality study might lead to a type 1 or type 2 error, further complicating the study results.[27] It is also apparent that there is not an effective, standardized way to assess RCT quality, and therefore evidence must be carefully measured.[28] One review found that half of the studies involving a particular topic did not fulfill the basic methodological standards for a high-quality study.[29]

There are other problems inherent with evidence-based medicine, including the emphasis it places on hierarchies (**Fig. 2**). This dependency might inadvertently influence physicians to make decisions based on underpowered or flawed RCTs and to overlook a high-quality observational study owing to its lower rank in the hierarchy. If evidence-based medicine is to drive guidelines, it needs to be augmented with rigorously performed and methodologically sound studies that would make it a more valid source of information for decision makers and physicians. Because of the central role of the RCT in evidence-based medicine, many of the problems with evidence-based medicine can be avoided at this stage of the system. One common problem involves the substantial variation in the results of many RCTs, including the fact that these studies often provide

contradictory results. Observational studies are known to be applicable in many areas, and Concato and colleagues[30] found that there was less variability in the results of these studies when compared with RCTs on the same topic. A study on the effectiveness of screening mammography documented that observational studies and RCTs yield similar estimates of efficacy, and that the case-control study is a valid source of evidence when performance of an RCT is not feasible.[31] In addition, observational studies can produce similar results to those of RCTs when using the same criteria in the selection of study subjects. In fact, one study found that on comparing RCTs and observational studies, one does not provide a consistently better effect than the other.[32]

We must be careful how we analyze and interpret studies before they are used to guide clinical decision-making policies. Physicians are becoming increasingly aware that the RCT is not the only form of valid study, and it is becoming clear that these studies must be performed in conjunction with observational studies to find the best evidence. Merkow and Ko[33] highlight the importance of using observational studies in a recent editorial, and how these types of studies may provide answers to clinical questions the RCT is not able to ascertain. Merkow and Ko looked specifically at a recent study by Giuliano and colleagues[34] that established an association between survival rates and metastases detected through the immunochemical staining of sentinel lymph nodes and bone marrow specimens from patients with early-stage breast cancer. The study was conducted to help resolve discrepancies in the variable evidence available from previously performed large retrospective studies on treatment, recurrence, survival rates, and recommendations regarding occult metastases. Using a series of statistical analyses, the investigators concluded that there is no valid clinical support for immunocytochemical examinations of bone marrow and immunohistochemical examinations of hematoxylin-eosin–negative sentinel lymph nodes for women with early-stage breast cancer. This study is a great example of a rigorously standardized, prospective cohort study that provides accurate and relevant evidence in cancer research for a subject that an RCT is not equipped to investigate.

Another major problem with the RCT is that by nature it excludes subjects in areas that are clinically relevant. RCTs often exclude complex multifaceted cases, or patients with a comorbidity that may have significant clinical importance. An RCT may also enroll a specific regulated population that is anticipated to be responsive to a particular type of treatment. In this situation, it might be

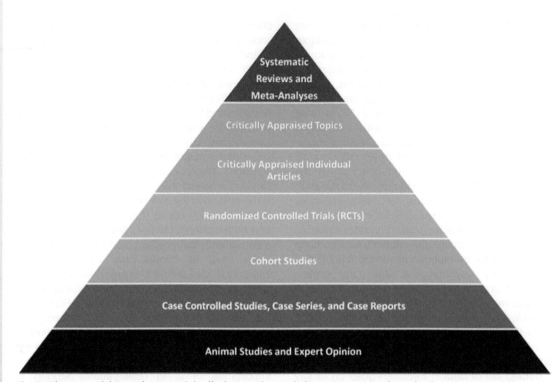

Fig. 2. The research hierarchy was originally designed to rank the various research methods so that it would be easier for the physician to translate the most relevant and valid data into the clinical setting. Although this hierarchy is a good representation of the levels of evidence for the different research methods, it should only be used as a guideline because evidence always needs to be independently evaluated before it is used to guide clinical decisions.

difficult for a physician to use this evidence and apply it to any patient who is not part of the group included in the study. For example, a potential RCT on breast reconstructive procedures after mastectomy may need to exclude patients who had prior radiation therapy because of the potential soft-tissue complications associated with implant-based reconstruction. Therefore, such exclusion criteria will not illuminate the outcomes of implant-based reconstruction for this common subset of patients who may benefit from a less extensive form of reconstructive technique. To combat the problems associated with evidence-based medicine we must educate medical professionals in its use, including what is considered credible and applicable evidence, how to properly conduct and analyze a systematic review and meta-analysis, and how to apply evidence to the clinical environment in a relevant way.

SUMMARY

The current state of health care reform calls for enhanced quality and decreased costs, and evidence-based medicine will be used to accomplish this goal. No matter the opinion of the individual physician on evidence-based medicine, it will increasingly dictate health care policy in the coming years. In fact, a recent poll in the *British Medical Journal* selected evidence-based medicine as 1 of the 15 greatest milestones in medicine since 1840, alongside medical advances such as antibiotics and vaccination. In addition, the recently enacted Patient Protection and Affordable Care Act will attempt to improve medical care by implementing "activities to improve patient safety and reduce medical errors through the appropriate use of best clinical practices, evidence-based medicine, and health information technology."[35] Despite its nearly universal acceptance and approval by numerous authorities, clinicians and academicians must remain diligent to prevent the abuse of evidence-based medicine, because as Alvan Feinstein said, "the threat of official, corporate, or private abuse will always remain."[26] As evidence-based medicine becomes a more important aspect of the medical industry, it is critical that all physicians learn how to properly conduct and use this novel approach to improving the quality of health care.

REFERENCES

1. Mountokalakis TD. Hippocrates and the essence of evidence based medicine. Hospital Chronicles 2006;1:7–8.

2. Aravind M, Chung KC. Evidence-based medicine and hospital reform: tracing origins back to Florence Nightingale. Plast Reconstr Surg 2010;125:403–9.

3. Kaska SC, Weinstein JN. Historical perspective. Ernest Amory Codman, 1869-1940. A pioneer of evidence-based medicine: the end result idea. Spine (Phila Pa 1976) 1998;23:629–33.

4. Greene AK, May JW Jr. Ernest Amory Codman, M.D. (1869 to 1940): the influence of the End Result Idea on plastic and reconstructive surgery. Plast Reconstr Surg 2007;119:1606–9.

5. Shah HM, Chung KC. Archie Cochrane and his vision for evidence-based medicine. Plast Reconstr Surg 2009;124:982–8.

6. Chassin MR, Brook RH, Park RE, et al. Variations in the use of medical and surgical services by the Medicare population. N Engl J Med 1986;314:285–90.

7. Wennberg J, Gittelsohn A. Small area variations in health care delivery. Science 1973;182:1102–8.

8. Stockwell H, Vayda E. Variations in surgery in Ontario. Med Care 1979;17:390–6.

9. Vayda E. A comparison of surgical rates in Canada and in England and Wales. N Engl J Med 1973;289:1224–9.

10. Roos NP, Roos LL. High and low surgical rates: risk factors for area residents. Am J Public Health 1981;71:591–600.

11. Haymart MR, Banerjee M, Stewart AK, et al. Use of radioactive iodine for thyroid cancer. JAMA 2011;306:721–8.

12. Roos NP, Roos LL Jr. Surgical rate variations: do they reflect the health or socioeconomic characteristics of the population? Med Care 1982;20:945–58.

13. Roos NP, Roos LL Jr, Henteleff PD. Elective surgical rates—do high rates mean lower standards? Tonsillectomy and adenoidectomy in Manitoba. N Engl J Med 1977;297:360–5.

14. LoGerfo JP. Variation in surgical rates: fact vs. fantasy. N Engl J Med 1977;297:387–9.

15. Roos NP, Henteleff PD, Roos LL Jr. A new audit procedure applied to an old question: is the frequency of T&A justified? Med Care 1977;15:1–18.

16. Lembcke PA. Measuring the quality of medical care through vital statistics based on hospital service areas; I. Comparative study of appendectomy rates. Am J Public Health Nations Health 1952;42:276–86.

17. Sackett DL, Haynes RB, Gibson ES, et al. Randomised clinical trial of strategies for improving medication compliance in primary hypertension. Lancet 1975;1:1205–7.

18. How to read clinical journals: I. why to read them and how to start reading them critically. Can Med Assoc J 1981;124:555–8.

19. Sur RL, Dahm P. History of evidence-based medicine. Indian J Urol 2011;27:487–9.

20. Guyatt G. Evidence-based medicine. ACP J Club (Ann Intern Med) 1991;114(Suppl 2):A–16.

21. Evidence-Based Medicine Working Group. Evidence-based medicine. A new approach to teaching the practice of medicine. JAMA 1992;268:2420–5.

22. Sackett DL, Rosenberg WM, Gray JA, et al. Evidence based medicine: what it is and what it isn't. BMJ 1996;312:71–2.

23. Guyatt GH, Haynes RB, Jaeschke RZ, et al. Users' Guides to the Medical Literature: XXV. Evidence-based medicine: principles for applying the Users' Guides to patient care. Evidence-Based Medicine Working Group. JAMA 2000;284:1290–6.

24. Montori VM, Guyatt GH. Progress in evidence-based medicine. JAMA 2008;300:1814–6.

25. Committee on Quality of Health Care in America IoM. Crossing the quality chasm: a new health system for the 21st century. Washington, DC: National Academic Press; 2001.

26. Feinstein AR, Horwitz RI. Problems in the "evidence" of "evidence-based medicine". Am J Med 1997;103:529–35.

27. Detsky AS, Naylor CD, O'Rourke K, et al. Incorporating variations in the quality of individual randomized trials into meta-analysis. J Clin Epidemiol 1992;45:255–65.

28. Moher D, Jadad AR, Nichol G, et al. Assessing the quality of randomized controlled trials: an annotated bibliography of scales and checklists. Control Clin Trials 1995;16:62–73.

29. Reid MC, Lachs MS, Feinstein AR. Use of methodological standards in diagnostic test research. Getting better but still not good. JAMA 1995;274:645–51.

30. Concato J, Shah N, Horwitz RI. Randomized, controlled trials, observational studies, and the hierarchy of research designs. N Engl J Med 2000;342:1887–92.

31. Demissie K, Mills OF, Rhoads GG. Empirical comparison of the results of randomized controlled trials and case-control studies in evaluating the effectiveness of screening mammography. J Clin Epidemiol 1998;51:81–91.

32. McKee M, Britton A, Black N, et al. Methods in health services research. Interpreting the evidence: choosing between randomised and non-randomised studies. BMJ 1999;319:312–5.

33. Merkow RP, Ko CY. Evidence-based medicine in surgery: the importance of both experimental and observational study designs. JAMA 2011;306:436–7.

34. Giuliano AE, Hawes D, Ballman KV, et al. Association of occult metastases in sentinel lymph nodes and bone marrow with survival among women with early-stage invasive breast cancer. JAMA 2011;306:385–93.

35. The Patient Protection and Affordable Care Act. In: Washington, DC: United States Congress; 2009. p. 1–2409.

Development and Psychometric Evaluation of the FACE-Q Satisfaction with Appearance Scale

A New Patient-Reported Outcome Instrument for Facial Aesthetics Patients

Andrea L. Pusic, MD, MD, MHS, FRCSC[a,*],
Anne F. Klassen, DPhil, BA[b], Amie M. Scott, MPH[a],
Stefan J. Cano, PhD[c]

KEYWORDS

- Facial cosmetic surgery • Aesthetic surgery • Outcomes • Quality of life • Patient satisfaction
- Psychometrics • Questionnaire • Rasch measurement

KEY POINTS

- Accurate and reliable measurement of patient-centered outcomes is critical to ongoing practice improvement and clinical research in facial aesthetics.
- Modern psychometric methods overcome the limitations of traditional psychometric methods by providing clinically meaningful interval-level data.
- The FACE-Q Satisfaction with Facial Appearance scale is a new-generation condition-specific patient-reported outcome instrument, capable of providing clinically meaningful and scientifically sound data reflecting patient perceptions of outcome.

BACKGROUND

Facial aesthetics procedures are an important area of continued growth in plastic surgery; 13.8 million cosmetic procedures were performed in the United States in 2011, an increase of 5% from 2010.[1] Rhinoplasty (n = 244,000) and blepharoplasty (n = 196,000) were second and third to breast augmentation (n = 307,000) in popularity.

Botulinum toxin type A (n = 5.7 million), soft tissue fillers (n = 1.9 million) and chemical peels (n = 1.1 million) were the top three cosmetic minimally invasive procedures.[1]

Specially designed questionnaires known as patient-reported outcome (PRO) instruments, developed to measure a range of outcomes (eg, symptoms, satisfaction, body image, and quality

Disclosure: The FACE-Q © is owned by Memorial Sloan-Kettering Cancer Center (MSKCC). Drs Cano, Klassen, and Pusic are codevelopers of the FACE-Q © and, as such, receive a share of any license revenues based on MSKCC's inventor sharing policy.
This study was funded by grants from the Plastic Surgery Education Foundation.
[a] Memorial Sloan-Kettering Cancer Center, Room MRI-1007, 1275 York Avenue, New York, NY 10065, USA;
[b] McMaster University, Department of Pediatrics, 3N27, 1280 Main Street W, Hamilton, ON L8S 4K1, Canada;
[c] Plymouth University Peninsula Schools of Medicine and Dentistry, Clinical Neurology Research Group, Tamar Science Park, Plymouth PL6 8BX, UK
* Corresponding author. Clinical Neurology Research Group, Plastic and Reconstructive Surgery, Memorial Sloan-Kettering Cancer Center, Tamar Science Park, Room MRI-1007, 1275 York Avenue, New York, NY 10065, USA.
E-mail address: pusica@mskcc.org

Clin Plastic Surg 40 (2013) 249–260
http://dx.doi.org/10.1016/j.cps.2012.12.001
0094-1298/13/$ – see front matter © 2013 Elsevier Inc. All rights reserved.

of life), have become a mainstay of clinical research in all areas of medicine and surgery.[2–4] To provide meaningful measurement, such PRO instruments must be shown to be reliable, valid, and responsive (**Table 1**).[2,5] Although understanding the patient's perspective is especially important in facial aesthetics, a systematic review performed by our team identified that there is a lack of reliable and valid PRO instruments available for measuring the range of issues important to facial aesthetic patients.[6] We therefore set out to develop a new PRO instrument following the methodology we previously used to develop other plastic surgery–specific PRO instruments.[7–9] This new PRO instrument is called the FACE-Q and includes a range of separate scales that measure important outcomes for patients having any type of facial cosmetic surgery, minimally invasive cosmetic procedure, or facial injectable.

This article describes the development and psychometric evaluation of the core FACE-Q scale, called the Satisfaction with Facial Appearance scale.

QUALITATIVE AND QUANTITATIVE METHODS

We obtained local institutional ethics review board approval before commencing our study. The content for the Satisfaction with Facial Appearance scale was developed as part of a larger suite of scales that cover a range of concepts important to facial aesthetics patients.[10] These scales were constructed with strict adherence to recommended guidelines for PRO instrument development.[11–15] The guidelines outline three phases required to develop a scientifically credible and clinically meaningful tool.

In the first phase, a conceptual framework is formally defined, and a pool of items is generated. These items are developed from the following three sources: review of the literature, qualitative patient interviews, and expert opinion. The item pool is developed into a series of scales that are pilot tested in the target participant sample to clarify ambiguities in item wording, confirm appropriateness, and determine acceptability and completion time. This phase of our research is described in a separate publication[10] and is summarized later in this paper. In the second phase (the main focus of this article), the scales undergo psychometric evaluation in a large sample of target subjects. Questions representing the best indicators of outcome are retained based on their performance against a standardized set of psychometric criteria. In the third phase, further psychometric evaluation is performed by administering the item-reduced scales to a large sample

of participants to further examine their scientific soundness.[16,17]

Phase 1: Qualitative Phase

Qualitative interviews were conducted with 50 patients recruited from 7 offices of plastic surgeons and dermatologists practicing in New York (United States) and Vancouver (Canada) between January 2008 and February 2009. Participants ranged in age from 20 to 79 years (mean age 51 years) and had undergone 1 or more of the following facial procedures: botulinum toxin (n = 20), resurfacing (n = 15), filler (n = 15), blepharoplasty (n = 25), facelift (n = 22), rhinoplasty (n = 9), neck lift (n = 8), brow lift (n = 4), and chin implant (n = 2).

Patients were interviewed using open-ended questions. Interviews were digitally recorded and transcribed verbatim and coded within NVivo8 software[18] using a line-by-line coding approach. Data collection and analysis took place concurrently to gather data to refine emerging codes and categories. Data analyses led to the development of a conceptual framework that depicts important concepts for facial aesthetic patients (**Fig. 1**).

To develop scales with items covering the concepts in **Fig. 1**, we examined codes (ie, key phrases expressed by patients) and linked these to specific patient characteristics (eg, type of procedure, age, and gender). Attaching key patient characteristics to each code provided the information needed to develop core items (common to all patients), and unique items (specific to a subgroup). To develop a set of scales, we then iteratively and interactively examined the item lists developed from the coded material to identify a set of items that mapped out a continuum for each major concept. For each item we examined Flesch-Kincaid grade level scores[19] and adjusted as necessary to ensure the lowest possible grade level for reading. Scale instructions and appropriate response options were then developed for each scale.

The scales were then presented to 26 experts (15 plastic surgeons, 4 dermatologists, 3 psychologists, 4 office staff) to further appraise and refine. In addition, 35 facial aesthetic patients participated in one-on-one cognitive debriefing interviews to identify any ambiguous wording and confirm appropriateness, acceptability, and completion time of the preliminary scales. The process resulted in the development of a set of independently functioning scales that measure the concepts forming the conceptual framework (**Table 2**).

Table 1
Glossary of terms

Term	Definition
Ad hoc questionnaire	A PRO instrument that has not been developed and/or validated using acknowledged guidelines.[6,17,49–51] Such PRO instruments may pose clinically reasonable questions, but one cannot be confident about their reliability (ie, ability to produce consistent and reproducible scores) or validity (ie, ability to measure what is intended to be measured)
Conceptual framework	The expected relationships of items within a domain and between domains within a PRO concept. The validation process confirms the conceptual framework
Domain	A domain is a collective word for a group of related concepts. All the items in a single domain contribute to the measurement of the domain concept
Generic questionnaires	PRO instruments that can be used in any patient group regardless of their health condition, and allow direct comparisons across disease groups and/or healthy populations. An example of a generic questionnaire is the Short Form 36-Item Health Survey, which is the most widely used generic measure in the world[52]
Health-related quality of life	In quality-of-life measurement, the terms quality of life, health status, health-related quality of life, and functional status are often used interchangeably. Although there is a lack of conceptual clarity regarding these terms,[53] there is broad agreement on the core minimum set of health concepts that should be measured.[54] These concepts include physical health, mental health, social functioning, role functioning, and general health perceptions
Item	An individual question, statement, or task that is evaluated by the patient to address a particular concept
PRO instrument	A questionnaire used in a clinical or research setting in which responses are collected directly from patients. These questionnaires quantify aspects of health-related quality of life and/or significant outcome variables (eg, patient satisfaction, symptoms) from the patient's perspective.[17] PRO instruments provide a means of quantifying the way patients perceive their health and the impact treatments have on their quality of life
Reliability	An important property of a PRO instrument because it is essential to establish that any changes observed in patient groups are attributable to the intervention or disease and not to problems in the measure. Test-retest reliability may be evaluated by having individuals complete a questionnaire on more than 1 occasion over a time period when no changes in outcome are expected to have occurred. Commonly reported reliability statistics include the Cronbach alpha[39] and intraclass correlation coefficients[16]
Responsiveness	The ability of an instrument to accurately detect change. Responsiveness is an important psychometric property when evaluating change as the result of a health care intervention or when following patients over time. Responsiveness is usually examined by comparing preintervention and postintervention scores using standardized change indicators, such as effect size statistics[41]
Scale	The system of numbers or verbal anchors by which a value or score is derived. Examples include visual analog scales, Likert scales, and rating scales
Scientific soundness	Refers to the demonstration of reliable, valid, and responsive measurement of the outcome of interest
Score	A number derived from a patient's response to items in a questionnaire. A score is computed based on a prespecified, validated scoring algorithm and is subsequently used in statistical analyses of clinical study results. Scores can be computed for individual items, domains, or concepts, or as a summary of items, domains, or concepts
Validity	The ability of an instrument to measure what is intended to be measured. Establishment of validity may be considered an ongoing process. A PRO instrument is examined from various angles, including an assessment of the development process, consideration of known group differences, evaluation of internal consistency, and evaluation of both convergent and discriminant validity relative to other existing related measures

Adapted from Food and Drug Administration. Patient reported outcome measures: use in medical product development to support labeling claims. 2009;11:31–3. Available at: www.fda.gov/cber/gdlns/prolbl.pdf; and Cano S, Klassen A, Pusic A. The science behind quality-of-life measurement: a primer for plastic surgeons. Plast Reconstr Surg 2009;123:99–102e; with permission.

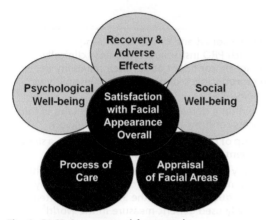

Fig. 1. FACE-Q conceptual framework.

Phase 2: Quantitative Phase

Data were collected and analyzed to identify the items representing the best indicators for each scale based on their performance against a standardized set of psychometric criteria. Data came from 2 separate studies, and were compiled for the purpose of psychometric analyses. Results presented in this article relate only to the Satisfaction with Facial Appearance scale. This scale was developed for use in research and clinical practice to compare outcomes across procedure types and/or to measure change before and after any facial aesthetic procedure. Future publications will present psychometric findings for the other FACE-Q scales.

Study 1

Data were collected from patients of 10 plastic surgeons and 2 dermatologists representing 10 different practices in the United States (New York, Washington, St Louis, Dallas, and Atlanta) and Canada (Vancouver) between June 2010 and June 2012. Eligible participants included those who could read English; were 18 years of age or older; and were planning to undergo, or had already undergone, any surgical or nonsurgical facial aesthetic procedure.

Given the large number of FACE-Q scales that were developed in the initial phases of research, we grouped scales into booklets based on common surgical and nonsurgical procedures and distributed these to the participating practices. All booklets included the Satisfaction with Facial Appearance scale. Instructions for this scale asked patients to answer a series of items based on "how you look right now" and to complete each item with their "entire face in mind." The 4 response options were as follows: very dissatisfied, somewhat dissatisfied, somewhat satisfied, and

Table 2 FACE-Q scales	
Appearance appraisal scales	Facial appearance overall[a],* Skin Lines overall Forehead lines Forehead and eyebrows Lines between eyebrows Eyes (overall, double eyelid, upper and lower eyelids) Crow's feet Eyelashes Cheekbones Cheeks Ears Nasal bridge Nose Nasolabial folds Lips Lip lines Marionette lines Chin Lower face/jawline Under Chin Neck
Quality of life scales*	Psychological wellbeing Social well-being Age appraisal Expectations and motivations Psychological distress Recovery early life impact*
Adverse effect checklists for treatment	Recovery early symptoms Skin Forehead, scalp and eyebrows Eyes Nose Lower face and neck Lips Ears
Process of care scales*	Decision Doctor Information Office staff Office appearance

[a] see **Table 4** for scale's content.
* Relevant scales for all patients.

very satisfied. Patient responses to items in each scale are converted to a summary score which ranges from 0 to 100. A higher score indicates higher satisfaction or better quality of life.

Patients from 6 surgical practices were recruited at the time of their appointment and asked to complete a questionnaire booklet in the waiting room before their appointment. Patients from 4 practices were invited to participate in a postal survey. To ensure a high response rate, a personalized letter from the relevant health care provider was included with the appropriate FACE-Q booklet and up to 3 mailed reminders were sent as necessary.[20,21] All patients invited into the study were given a gift card ($5) to thank them for their participation.

Study 2

A medical device company was provided with the Satisfaction with Facial Appearance scale alongside other FACE-Q scales relevant to measuring the concerns of patients having facelifts for a clinical trial involving 100 patients from France, Germany, the United Kingdom, and Israel. Patients completed FACE-Q scales before and after surgery. MAPI (MArchés et Prospectives Internationaux [International Prospects and Markets in English]) Research Trust[22] provided translations and linguistic validation of the FACE-Q scales. This process ensured that the concepts measured by the FACE-Q scales are equivalent across languages (ie, English, German, French, and Hebrew) and easily understood by the people in the target country. In brief, MAPI uses a process based on translation principles as detailed by the European Regulatory Issues and Quality of Life Assessment (ERIQA) group[23] and the International Society of Pharmacoeconomics and Outcomes Research[24,25] and recommended by the US Food and Drug Administration.[11]

Rasch measurement theory and analysis We analyzed the Satisfaction with Facial Appearance scale data using Rasch measurement theory methods.[26,27] These methods are increasingly used in health outcome research.[28] Unlike traditional methods, Rasch analysis indicates the extent to which rigorous measurement is achieved by examining the difference (or fit) between the observed scores (patients' responses to items) and the expected values predicted from the data by a single mathematical model called the Rasch model. The criteria for measurement in Rasch analysis are evaluated interactively using the Rasch model.[29,30] Thus, a range of evidence is used to evaluate each questionnaire item in a scale. This evidence is then used to make a judgment about the overall quality of the scale.

Rasch analyses were performed on the Satisfaction with Facial Appearance scale using RUMM2030 software.[31] Results were interpreted using published criteria wherever possible as follows:

Item fit validity The items of the Satisfaction with Facial Appearance scale must work together (fit) as a conformable set both clinically and statistically. When items do not work together (misfit) in this way, it is inappropriate to sum item responses to reach a total score, and the validity of a scale is questioned. Three main indicators were examined to assess item fit[27,29]:

1. Log residuals (item-person interaction)
2. Chi-square values (item-trait interaction)
3. Item characteristic curves

There are no absolute criteria for interpreting fit statistics. It is more meaningful to interpret them together and in the context of their clinical usefulness as an item set. However, as a guide, fit residual should be between -2.5 and $+2.5$ with associated nonsignificant chi-square values (significance interpreted after Bonferroni adjustment).

Each of the items of the Satisfaction with Facial Appearance scale has multiple response categories (ie, very dissatisfied, somewhat dissatisfied, somewhat satisfied and very satisfied), which reflect an ordered continuum. Although this ordering may seem clinically sensible at the item level, it must also work together when the items are combined to form a set. Item fit validity analysis tests this statistically and graphically by threshold locations and plots. As such, the threshold values between adjacent pairs of response options for each item are expected to be ordered by magnitude (less to more). Thresholds are visible in graphical plots, in which the highest areas of the probability distributions of each response category should not be below adjacent category plots. When response options work as expected, important evidence for the validity of the scale is obtained.[32]

Targeting Scale-to-sample targeting concerns the match between the range of satisfaction with facial appearance measured by the Satisfaction with Facial Appearance items and the range of satisfaction with facial appearance as reported by a sample of patients. Targeting can be observed by examining the spread of person and item locations (ie, define the relative distributions of transformed total scores against the locations of the individual items across the continuum of satisfaction with facial appearance) in these two relative distributions. Targeting analysis informs about how suitable the sample is for evaluating the Satisfaction with Facial Appearance scale and how suitable the scale is for measuring the sample. Better targeting equates to a better ability to interpret the psychometric data with confidence.[27,33]

Reliability Person measurements (estimates) are examined with the Person Separation Index (PSI), a reliability statistic that is comparable with the Cronbach alpha.[34] The PSI quantifies the error associated with the measurements of people in a sample. Higher PSI values indicate better reliability (>0.70 indicates adequate reliability[33]).

Stability Scale performance (specifically item performance) should be stable across clinically important scenarios in which systematic differences between subgroups that may lead to bias in responding to items are not expected. Stability analysis enables an explicit test of scale performance in the form of an examination of differential item functioning (DIF). We examined DIF for gender, age, and ethnicity. As a guide, statistically significant chi-square values indicate potential DIF and therefore problems in scale performance (significance interpreted after Bonferroni adjustment).[35]

Traditional psychometric methods analysis Traditional psychometric methods primarily use correlation or descriptive analyses to evaluate scaling assumptions (legitimacy of summing items) and scale reliability and validity, which are described in detail elsewhere.[33] We examined data quality (percent missing data for

calculating half standard deviation of the pretreatment mean score, and (2) extrapolation of a change score based on a 0.5 ES.

The responsiveness of the Satisfaction with Facial Appearance scale was also compared at the individual person level. This change score was achieved by computing, for each person, the significance of their own change in measurement (sig change).[43] First, we computed a change score for each person (before surgery to after surgery). Second, we computed the standard error associated with each person's change score (ie, the square root of the sum of the squared standard error values before and after surgery). Third, we computed the significance of the change for each person by dividing their change score by the standard error of the difference (SE_{diff}; ie, how large was their change in standard error units). Fourth, we categorized the significance of each person's change score into 1 of 5 groups according to the size and direction of the change score. We then counted the numbers of people achieving each level of significance of change. The formulae are as follows:

$$\text{Sig change} = \frac{\text{Postsurgery transformed score} - \text{Presurgery transformed score}}{SE_{diff}}$$

where SE_{diff} for a person $= \sqrt{(\text{SE presurgery transformed score})^2 + (\text{SE postsurgery transformed score})^2}$

each item), scaling assumptions (similarity of item means and variances; magnitude and similarity of corrected item-total correlations[36–38]), scale-to-sample targeting (score means; standard deviation [SD]; floor and ceiling effects), and internal consistency reliability (Cronbach alpha,[39] homogeneity coefficients[40]).

Responsiveness analysis The responsiveness of the Satisfaction with Facial Appearance scale to detect clinical change was examined in the largest subgroup in our sample (patients having facelifts) at the group level by comparing pretreatment and posttreatment Rasch transformed scores using paired *t*-tests and calculating the following 2 standard indicators: effect size (ES) calculations (Kazis ES[41]); and standardized response mean (SRM).[42] Larger ESs/SRMs indicate greater responsiveness, and it is standard practice to interpret the magnitude of the change using Cohen arbitrary criteria (0.20, small; 0.50, moderate; and 0.80, large). Preliminary minimal importance difference (MID) values were generated as follows: (1)

Significance of change values obtained from this formula was categorized into the following 5 groups:

Significant improvement = Sig change $\geq$ +1.96
Nonsignificant improvement = 0 < Sig Change $\leq$ +1.95
No change = Sig change = 0
Nonsignificant worsening = $-1.95 \leq$ Sig change < 0
Significant worsening = Sig change $\leq$ −1.96

RESULTS
Phase 1: Qualitative Phase

As described earlier and in our previous publication,[10] the qualitative work resulted in the development of a conceptual framework (see **Fig. 1**) and a series of independent scales that capture the important concerns described by facial aesthetics patients (see **Table 2**). The Satisfaction with Facial Appearance scale was specifically developed to be relevant to all aesthetic facial patients regardless of the number or type of procedures undergone. This scale is composed of 10 items that ask about satisfaction using descriptors (eg, symmetry, balance, proportion) as well as scenarios (eg, in photographs, under bright lights). The item set is easy to understand and complete with a Flesch Kincaid grade level of 0.8, and all items lower than grade 6 (range 0–5.2).

Phase 2: Quantitative Phase

A total of 360 patients were invited to participate through face-to-face recruitment, and 332 responded. A further 283 patients were sent the FACE-Q in the mail, and 167 responded. The overall response rate was 78%. Participants ranged in age from 18 to 85 years; 64 were men and 409 were women (**Table 3**). Participants completed from 1 to 3 copies of the FACE-Q at various time points.

Rasch analyses
Overall, the results of Rasch analysis supported the Satisfaction with Facial Appearance scale as a reliable and valid measure of satisfaction with facial appearance. All 10 items had ordered thresholds, which supports the appropriateness of the number and type of response options we created (**Fig. 2**). Just 1 of the 10 items had fit residuals marginally outside of the −2.5 to +2.5 range (Q4). However, no item had a significant chi-square value (**Table 4**). Distributions of item thresholds and person estimates were well matched, taking into consideration some gaps at the extremes of the continuum (lowest/highest satisfaction) (**Fig. 3**). The PSI was 0.92, showing good reliability. Analysis of the data set showed no statistical DIF by gender, age, or ethnicity (**Table 5**).

Traditional psychometric analysis
The results of traditional analysis also supported the Satisfaction with Facial Appearance scale as a reliable and valid measure (**Table 6**). The criteria were satisfied for all psychometric properties evaluated. Data quality was high (missing data range ≤2%, scale scores were computable for 98% of respondents) and scaling assumptions were satisfied (similar mean item scores, corrected item-total correlations range = 0.75–0.82). Scale-to-sample targeting was good (scale scores spanned the scale range and were not notably skewed; the scale midpoint, and ceiling effects were negligible), and internal consistency reliability was high (Cronbach alpha = 0.95; mean item-item correlation = 0.65 [0.52–0.89]).

Table 3 Patient characteristics from field tests		
	Study 1	Study 2
N	399	100
Age (y)		
Mean (SD)	48.9 (14.8)	54.3 (7.8)
Range	18–85	37–77
Gender		
Female (%)	323 (85.7)	86 (89.6)
Male (%)	54 (14.3)	10 (10.4)
Ethnicity		
White non-Hispanic (%)	269 (73.5)	100 (100)
Asian (%)	21 (5.8)	—
South Asian (%)	18 (4.9)	—
Native American (%)	17 (4.6)	—
White Hispanic (%)	13 (3.6)	—
Black non-Hispanic (%)	10 (2.7)	—
Other (%)	18 (4.9)	—
Country		
United States (%)	197 (49.5)	—
Canada (%)	201 (50.5)	—
France (%)	—	15 (15)
Germany (%)	—	50 (50)
Israel (%)	—	20 (20)
United Kingdom (%)	—	15 (15)
Timing of Booklet		
Before only (%)	61(15.3)	12 (12)
After only (%)	294 (73.6)	—
Before and 1 after (%)	26 (6.5)	88 (88)
Before and 2 after (%)	9 (2.3)	—
2 after only	9 (2.3)	—
Booklet Type		
Fillers (%)	57 (14.2)	—
Botulinum toxin (%)	75 (18.8)	—
Skin resurfacing (%)	17 (4.3)	—
Lip injections (%)	11 (2.8)	—
Facelift (%)	97 (24.3)	100 (100)
Blepharoplasty (%)	65 (16.3)	—
Rhinoplasty (%)	45 (11.3)	—
Chin surgery (%)	22 (5.5)	—
Brow lift (%)	4 (1.0)	—
Cheeks (%)	6 (1.5)	—

Responsiveness
Group-level findings Ninety-seven patients completed presurgery and 6-month postsurgery versions of the scale. The responsiveness data generated by the analysis of interval measurements showed that the scale quantified significant change

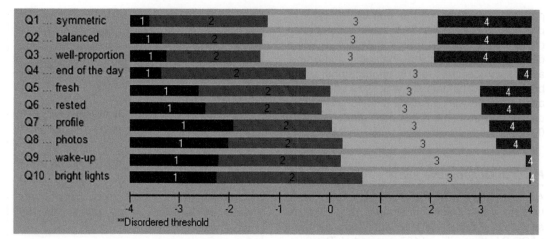

Fig. 2. Ordering of item response thresholds (location order). Threshold map for all items in the FACE-Q Satisfaction with Facial Appearance scale. The x-axis symbolizes the construct (satisfaction with facial appearance), with satisfaction increasing to the right. The y-axis shows the items' response categories: 1, very unsatisfied (*blue block*); 2, somewhat dissatisfied (*red block*); 3, somewhat satisfied (*green block*); 4, very satisfied (*purple block*).

at the group level. Patients' satisfaction with their facial appearance on a 0–100 scale was significantly higher following facelift-related treatment than it was before treatment (mean, SD = 45, 16 vs 56, 21, respectively, $P<.0001$). These statistically significant change scores were associated with moderate effect sizes (ES = 0.68, SRM = 0.50). In addition, preliminary MID analyses suggested an 8-point difference in total scores. This difference was exceeded in our analysis (mean change, SD = 11, 22).

Individual-level findings 94 out of 97 patients who had facelifts reported significant improvement in satisfaction with facial appearance, with the remaining 3 patients reporting nonsignificant

improvement. This finding supports the scale's ability to measure important change following treatment.

DISCUSSION

Satisfaction with appearance and improved quality of life are arguably the most important outcomes for patients undergoing facial aesthetic procedures.[4,44] Despite this, research in facial aesthetics has been hindered by a lack of reliable and valid condition-specific PRO instruments. The FACE-Q is developed to address this void. In this study, the FACE-Q Satisfaction with Facial Appearance scale is a short, easy to complete, reliable, valid and responsive measurement tool.

Table 4
Statistical indicators of fit (fit residual; chi-square)

	Items	Item Location	SE	Fit Residual	Chi-Square	P
Q1	...symmetric	−0.91	0.08	0.26	3.53	.474
Q2	...balanced	−0.86	0.08	−2.21	7.15	.128
Q3	...well proportioned	−0.85	0.08	−0.79	9.44	.051
Q4	...end of day[a]	−0.03	0.08	−2.59	10.56	.032
Q5	...fresh	0.13	0.08	−1.66	4.77	.311
Q6	...rested	0.13	0.08	−1.64	8.03	.090
Q7	...profile	0.44	0.07	0.93	3.83	.430
Q8	...photos	0.51	0.07	1.75	3.80	.433
Q9	...wake-up	0.64	0.08	0.59	0.88	.927
Q10	...bright lights	0.80	0.08	−2.01	7.58	.108

Items are in serial order.
Abbreviation: SE, standard error.
[a] Fit residual outside + 2.5 criteria.

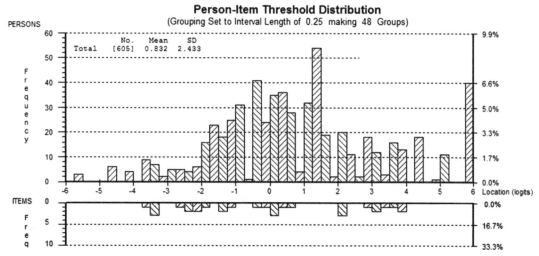

Fig. 3. Targeting of scale to sample (person-item threshold locations spread). The x-axis symbolizes the construct (satisfaction with facial appearance), with satisfaction increasing to the right. The y-axis shows the frequency of person measure locations (*top histogram*) and item locations (*bottom histogram*).

Our study provides the first empirical support for the use of this scale to measure satisfaction in patients undergoing any type of surgical or non-surgical facial aesthetic procedure.

There are several strengths to this research. The FACE-Q Satisfaction with Facial Appearance scale was developed from qualitative research that involved in-depth interviews with a varied sample of patients as well as extensive expert input.[10] Careful qualitative work was instrumental to establishing a strong conceptual framework and a valid set of scales with items capable of measuring the unique concerns of patients having facial aesthetic surgery. Thus, unlike generic PRO instruments that have been used in plastic surgery studies in the past, our Satisfaction with Facial Appearance scale is well calibrated to measure preprocedure to postprocedure change. As a further strength, psychometric evaluation of the Satisfaction with Facial Appearance scale involved a large heterogeneous patient sample and our DIF results indicate that the scale performed the same in subgroups of patients that varied by age, gender, and ethnicity.

Accurate and reliable quantification of patient-centered outcomes is critical to ongoing practice improvement and technical advancement in facial plastic surgery. Such quantification requires the use of high-quality PRO instruments that accurately measure patients' subjective perception of

Table 5
DIF: gender, age, and ethnicity

		Gender			Age			Ethnicity		
		MS	F	P	MS	F	P	MS	F	P
Q1	...symmetric	2.12	2.25	.135	1.31	1.42	.197	1.29	1.41	.210
Q2	...balanced	0.00	0.00	.994	2.25	2.99	.005	0.71	0.95	.462
Q3	...well proportioned	0.94	1.04	.309	1.93	2.14	.038	0.83	0.95	.458
Q4	...end of day	0.05	0.07	.792	1.14	1.53	.155	0.53	0.73	.629
Q5	...fresh	0.78	0.95	.330	0.93	1.12	.348	1.14	1.41	.208
Q6	...rested	0.13	0.15	.696	1.36	1.64	.123	0.40	0.47	.827
Q7	...profile	0.61	0.63	.428	0.55	0.56	.786	1.20	1.20	.305
Q8	...photographs	1.23	1.19	.276	2.18	2.16	.037	1.01	0.98	.442
Q9	...wake-up	0.03	0.03	.859	0.71	0.74	.640	0.29	0.30	.938
Q10	...bright lights	0.56	0.68	.410	2.24	2.82	.007	1.22	1.50	.175

Abbreviations: F, F-statistic; MS, mean square.

Table 6
Data quality, scaling assumptions, and targeting

| | | Data Quality | Scaling Assumptions | | | | | Targeting | |
		Item Missing Data (%)	Possible Range (Midpoint)	Score Range	Mean Score	SD	CITC	Floor/ Ceiling Effects (%)[a]	Skewness
Q1	...symmetric	1	1–4	1–4	3.07	0.80	0.75	4/32	−0.58
Q2	...balanced	1	1–4	1–4	3.08	0.82	0.78	5/33	−0.66
Q3	...well proportioned	1	1–4	1–4	3.09	0.82	0.77	5/33	−0.70
Q4	...end of day	1	1–4	1–4	2.82	0.82	0.81	6/20	−0.32
Q5	...fresh	1	1–4	1–4	2.78	0.91	0.82	9/25	−0.23
Q6	...rested	1	1–4	1–4	2.79	0.92	0.81	9/25	−0.29
Q7	...profile	2	1–4	1–4	2.71	0.94	0.78	12/22	−0.24
Q8	...photographs	2	1–4	1–4	2.67	0.93	0.75	12/21	−0.17
Q9	...wake-up	1	1–4	1–4	2.65	0.89	0.77	11/18	−0.17
Q10	...bright lights	2	1–4	1–4	2.59	0.90	0.81	11/17	−0.04
Total		2	10–40	10–40	28.3	7.3	—	1/8	−0.18

Abbreviation: CITC, corrected item-total correlation.
[a] Calculated as the percentage of people scoring either floor or ceiling.

outcomes and provide clinically meaningful interval-level data. Interval-level means that the scores derived from the FACE-Q Satisfaction with Facial Appearance scale have defined units and that the distance between each unit is the same.[45] Such interval-level measurement is analogous to measurements used in clinical practice, such as temperature in Celsius or millimeters on a ruler used in the operating room.[46]

The ability to move beyond raw scores to linearized measures is one of the benefits of Rasch measurement methods. Previous PRO instruments developed using traditional psychometric methods provide ordinal rather than interval-level measurement and, as such, have inherently limited clinical meaning. As an example, the Derriford scale is an older-generation PRO instrument developed to measure quality of life among patients having aesthetic surgery and developed using traditional methods providing only ordinal-level measurement. When a patient moves from a score of 100 to 120 on the Derriford scale following surgery, improvement has occurred; however, when another patient moves from 120 to 140, it cannot be assumed that both patients experienced the same magnitude of improvement from a 20-point change in score.[47] The FACE-Q is an example of a new generation of PRO instruments that can overcome the limitations of older-generation measures and provides clinical meaningful outcomes data. The advantages of

Rasch measurement theory in PRO instrument development include the ability to compare directly patients' total scores and the item locations on the same metric; the improved potential to diagnose item-level psychometric problems; and the ability to move to a more accurate picture of individual person measurements derived from PRO instruments.[48]

Our current study has 3 main limitations. First, in both our development and psychometric evaluation of the FACE-Q, most patients were female. Although this mirrors the patient population seen in clinical practice (and DIF analysis indicated that item performance was stable across genders), future research to explore the psychometric properties of the scale when used with male patients is warranted. Second, our sample included patients who may have had multiple procedures (both surgical and nonsurgical). Although this reflects real-world practice, and hence increases the validity of our findings, the impact of specific procedures in this particular study cannot confidently be delineated. In future clinical trials with stringent inclusion criteria, the impact of specific procedures on patient satisfaction and quality of life may be examined. Third, there is a potential for selection bias in our research. Although our response rate was high among patients who received the questionnaire while in clinic, it was lower when administered by mail and this may contribute to bias. In addition, practices where clinicians volunteer to recruit patients for PRO research may be different from practices that do not volunteer, and we did not have control over which patients the office staff recruited into the study.

The FACE-Q Satisfaction with Facial Appearance scale is an example of a new-generation condition-specific PRO instrument capable of providing highly reliable, valid, and responsive patient assessments. The scale has strong psychometric properties and the potential to provide clinically meaningful scores. By providing scientifically sound and clinical interpretable outcomes data, this scale (and others in the FACE-Q PRO instrument suite) will be able to inform technical advancement and ongoing practice improvement in future studies and in individual clinical care.

ACKNOWLEDGMENTS

The authors acknowledge and thank the following clinicians for their invaluable assistance with the recruitment of patients and countless hours spent as expert reviewers: Vancouver, BC, Canada: Drs Nick Carr, Francis Jang, Nancy VanLaeken, Alistair Carruthers, Jean Carruthers, Richard Warren. Washington DC: Dr Stephen Baker; Dallas, TX: Drs Jeffery Kenkel, Rod Rohrich; Atlanta GA: Dr Foad Nahai; St Louis, MO: Dr Leroy Young; New York, NY: Drs David Hidalgo, David Rosenberg, Philip Miller, Alexes Hazen, and Haideh Hirmand.

REFERENCES

1. American Society for Aesthetic Plastic Surgery. 2012. Available at: http://www.plasticsurgery.org/News-and-Resources/2011-Statistics-.html. Accessed Sept 21, 2012.

2. Pusic A, Lemaine V, Klassen A, et al. Patient-reported outcome measures in plastic surgery: use and interpretation in evidence-based medicine. Plast Reconstr Surg 2011;127:6.

3. Fitzpatrick R, Jenkinson C, Klassen A, et al. Methods of assessing health-related quality of life and outcome for plastic surgery. Br J Plast Surg 1999; 52:251–5.

4. Cano S, Browne J, Lamping D. Patient-based measures of outcome in plastic surgery: current approaches and future directions. Br J Plast Surg 2004;57:1–11.

5. Cano S, Hobart J. The problem with health measurement. Patient Prefer Adherence 2011;5:279–90.

6. Kosowski T, McCarthy C, Reavey P, et al. A systematic review of patient-reported outcome measures after facial cosmetic surgery and/or nonsurgical facial rejuvenation. Plast Reconstr Surg 2009;123:1819–27.

7. Cano S, Klassen A, Scott A, et al. The BREAST-Q ©: further validation in independent clinical samples. Plast Reconstr Surg 2012;129:293–302.

8. Klassen A, Pusic A, Scott A, et al. Satisfaction and quality of life in women who undergo breast surgery: a qualitative study. BMC Womens Health 2009;9:11–8.

9. Pusic A, Klassen A, Scott A, et al. Development of a new patient-reported outcome measure for breast surgery: the BREAST-Q. Plast Reconstr Surg 2009; 124:345–53.

10. Klassen A, Cano S, Scott A, et al. Measuring patient-reported outcomes in facial aesthetic patients: development of the FACE-Q. Facial Plast Surg 2010;26:303–9.

11. Food and Drug Administration. Patient reported outcome measures: use in medical product development to support labeling claims. 2009. Available at: www.fda.gov/cber/gdlns/prolbl.pdf. Accessed Sept 21, 2012.

12. Cano S, Hobart J. Watch out, watch out, the FDA are about. Dev Med Child Neurol 2008;50:108–9.

13. Mokkink L, Terwee C, Patrick D, et al. The COSMIN checklist for assessing the methodological quality of studies on measurement properties of health status measurement instruments: an international Delphi study. Qual Life Res 2010;19:539–49.

14. Scientific Advisory Committee of the Medical Outcomes Trust. Assessing health status and quality of life instruments: attributes and review criteria. Qual Life Res 2002;11:193–205.

15. Lasch K, Marquis P, Vigneuz M, et al. PRO development: rigorous qualitative research as crucial foundation. Qual Life Res 2010;19:9.

16. Hays R, Anderson R, Revicki D. Psychometric considerations in evaluating health-related quality of life measures. Qual Life Res 1993;2:441–9.

17. Cano S, Klassen A, Pusic A. The science behind quality-of-life measurement: a primer for plastic surgeons. Plast Reconstr Surg 2009;123:98e–106e.

18. Qualitative Solutions Research International: NVivo 8. Australia: QSR International; 2008.

19. Flesch R. A new readability yardstick. J Appl Psychol 1948;32:12.

20. Dillman D. Mail and telephone surveys: the total design method. New York: Wiley; 1978.

21. Dillman D. Mail and internet surveys: the tailored design method. 2nd edition. Toronto: Wiley; 2000.

22. MAPI Research Trust: France. 2004-2012. Available at: http://www.mapitrust.org/. Accessed Sept 21, 2012.

23. Chassany O, Sagnier P, Marquis P, et al. Patient-reported outcomes: the example of health-related quality of life — A European guidance document for the improved integration of health-related quality of

life assessment in the drug regulatory process. DIA J 2002;36:209–38.

24. Wild D, Grove A, Martin M, et al. Principles of good practice for the translation and cultural adaptation process for patient-reported outcomes (PRO) measures: report of the ISPOR Task Force for Translation and Cultural Adaptation. Value Health 2005;8: 94–104.

25. Wild D, Eremenco S, Mear I, et al. Multinational trials-recommendations on the translations required, approaches to using the same language in different countries, and the approaches to support pooling the data: the ISPOR Patient-Reported Outcomes Translation and Linguistic Validation Good Research Practices Task Force report. Value Health 2009; 12(4):430–40.

26. Andrich D. Controversy and the Rasch model: a characteristic of incompatible paradigms? Med Care 2004;42:17–116.

27. Wright B, Masters G. Rating scale analysis: Rasch measurement. Chicago: MESA; 1982.

28. Massof R. Understanding Rasch and item response theory models: applications to the estimation and validation of interval latent trait measures from responses to rating scale questionnaires. Ophthalmic Epidemiol 2011;18:19.

29. Andrich D. Rasch models for measurement. Beverley Hills (CA): Sage Publications; 1988.

30. Rasch G. Probabilistic models for some intelligence and attainment tests. Copenhagen (Denmark): Danish Institute for Education Research; 1960.

31. Andrich D, Sheridan B. RUMM 2030. Perth (Australia): RUMM Laboratory; 1997–2011.

32. Andrich D. Rating scales and Rasch measurement. Expert Rev Pharmacoecon Outcomes Res 2011; 11:14.

33. Hobart J, Cano S. Improving the evaluation of therapeutic intervention in MS: the role of new psychometric methods. Health Technol Assess 2009;13:1–200.

34. Andrich D. An index of person separation in latent trait theory, the traditional KR20 index and the Guttman scale response pattern. Educ Psychol Res 1982;9:9.

35. Hagquist C, Andrich D. Is the Sense of Coherence instrument applicable on adolescents? A latent trait analysis using Rasch modelling. Pers Indiv Differ 2004;36:13.

36. McHorney C, Haley S, Ware JJ. Evaluation of the MOS SF-36 Physical Functioning Scale (PF-10): II. Comparison of relative precision using Likert and Rasch scoring methods. J Clin Epidemiol 1997;50: 451–61.

37. Likert R. A technique for the measurement of attitudes. Arch Psychol 1932;140:50.

38. Ware J, Harris W, Gandek B, et al. MAP-R for Windows: multi-trait/multi-item analysis program—

revised user's guide. Boston: Health Assessment Laboratory; 1997.

39. Cronbach L. Coefficient alpha and the internal structure of tests. Psychometrika 1951;16:297–334.

40. Eisen M, Ware JJ, Donald C, et al. Measuring components of children's health status. Med Care 1979;17:19.

41. Kazis L, Anderson J, Meenan R. Effect sizes for interpreting changes in health status. Med Care 1989;27:178–89.

42. Liang M, Fossel A, Larson M. Comparisons of five health status instruments for orthopedic evaluation. Med Care 1990;28:10.

43. Hobart J, Cano S, Thompson A. Effect sizes can be misleading: is it time to change the way we measure change? J Neurol Neurosurg Psychiatry 2010;81:4.

44. Ching S, Thoma A, McCabe R, et al. Measuring outcomes in aesthetic surgery: a comprehensive review of the literature. Plast Reconstr Surg 2003; 111:11.

45. Wright B, Linacre J. Observations are always ordinal: measurements, however, must be interval. Arch Phys Med Rehabil 1989;70:857–60.

46. Bond T, Fox C. Applying the Rasch model. Fundamental measurement in the human sciences. 2nd edition. Mahwah, New Jersey: Lawrence Erlbaum Associates; 2007.

47. Harris D, Carr A. The Derriford Appearance Scale (DAS59): a new psychometric scale for the evaluation of patients with disfigurements and aesthetic problems of appearance. Br J Plast Surg 2001;54: 216–22.

48. Wright B. Solving measurement problems with the Rasch model. J Educ Meas 1977;14:97–116.

49. Branski R, Cukier-Blaj S, Pusic A, et al. Measuring quality of life in dysphonic patients: a systematic review of content development in patient-reported outcomes measures. J Voice 2010;24:193–8.

50. Klassen A, Stotland M, Skarsgard E, et al. Clinical research in pediatric plastic surgery and systematic review of quality-of-life questionnaires. Clin Plast Surg 2008;35:251–67.

51. Pusic A, Chen CM, Cano S, et al. Measuring quality of life in cosmetic and reconstructive breast surgery: a systematic review of patient-reported outcomes instruments. Plast Reconstr Surg 2007;120:823–37 [discussion: 838–9].

52. Garratt A, Schmidt L, Mackintosh A, et al. Quality of life measurement: bibliographic study of patient assessed health outcome measures. BMJ 2002;324: 1417.

53. Hunt S. The problem of quality of life. Qual Life Res 1997;6:205–12.

54. Lamping D. Methods for measuring outcomes to evaluate interventions to improve health-related quality of life in HIV. Psychol Health 1994;9:31–9.

How to Use Outcomes Questionnaires: Pearls and Pitfalls

Sunitha Malay, MPH, Kevin C. Chung, MD, MS*

KEYWORDS

- Patient-reported outcomes • Psychometric properties
- Generic and specific outcomes questionnaires

KEY POINTS

- If well-developed and validated tools are available for a condition, there is little need to develop new questionnaires except when they are simpler or provide enhanced information.
- Future efforts should focus on enabling the process of data collection and analysis through questionnaires simple enough to facilitate the regular use of these tools in clinical practice.
- In the current era of outcomes assessment and evidence-based medicine, it is essential for plastic surgeons to keep well-informed about the latest developments in understanding the assessment tools available to achieve enhanced patient satisfaction and quality of care.

OVERVIEW

Outcomes assessment is an integral component of evaluating the success of various medical and surgical procedures in the evidence-based era. Rather than relying on traditional "hard" outcomes data, such as how far one can walk after lower leg reconstruction or how much breast tissue is resected in breast reduction surgery, physicians and patients are much more interested in patients' perception of their functional improvement, quality of life, and satisfaction with treatment. Such appraisal is vital not only for clinicians but also to patients. Patients are constantly trying to derive maximum information from their surgeon with regard to the outcomes of the procedures they undergo. These inquiries extend farbeyond recovery and functional restoration. In plastic surgery, patients want to be reassured of other critical aspects of care, such as satisfaction, physical and social well-being, and aesthetic appearances as a result of an intervention.

Traditionally, outcomes are measured in the form of assessments made by the treating plastic surgeon through photographs, anatomic measurements, and complications. However, the perception of results by a surgeon and patient differ. A plastic surgeon may be content with the results obtained from his or her treatment, but the patient may not be similarly pleased with the outcomes achieved. Therefore, outcomes measured from the patient's viewpoint are highly relevant because most of the procedures performed in plastic surgery aim at improving physical appearance, body image, psychosocial function, and quality of life.[1] Acceptance by friends and family, emotional and mental satisfaction, confidence, and happiness with appearance after an intervention influence quality-of-life outcomes.[2] The volume of plastic surgery procedures is huge, and ever increasing.

Supported in part by grants from the National Institute on Aging and National Institute of Arthritis and Musculoskeletal and Skin Diseases (R01 AR062066) and from the National Institute of Arthritis and Musculoskeletal and Skin Diseases (2R01 AR047328-06) and a Midcareer Investigator Award in Patient-Oriented Research (K24 AR053120) (to Dr Kevin C. Chung).
Section of Plastic Surgery, Department of Surgery, The University of Michigan Health System, 1500 East Medical Center Drive, 2130 Taubman Center, SPC 5340, Ann Arbor, MI 48109–0340, USA
* Corresponding author.
E-mail address: kecchung@med.umich.edu

Procedural statistics from the American Society of Plastic Surgeons showed that 5.5 million reconstruction procedures and 1.6 million cosmetic surgical procedures were performed in the year 2011 with an increase of 5% and 2%, respectively, over the year 2010.[3] Therefore, subsequent assessment of outcomes from the patient's perspective is relevant in plastic surgery.

Measures to quantify the results in plastic surgery are a recent trend and in the last two decades several outcomes questionnaires or surveys in the form of patient-reported outcomes (PRO) were developed and used. However, all of these outcomes tools are not validated. Encouragingly, the last decade has seen much progress in this area and attempts to develop more robust measurement tools continue. Plastic surgery is a unique field in which outcomes are not assessed alone by mortality and morbidity. Therefore, patient satisfaction and quality-of-life components take prime importance.[2] The future and success of this specialty depends heavily on the patients' perception of their outcomes. The ultimate goal is to have outcomes measures that incorporate patient satisfaction and all of the quality-of-life measures that can potentially reflect the real effect of a surgical intervention. This article educates readers about how to use these tools to measure patient satisfaction and outcomes achieved in a more meaningful and coherent manner. It also informs readers about the common pearls and pitfalls encountered during use of these questionnaires.

PATIENT REPORTED OUTCOMES MEASUREMENT INFORMATION SYSTEM AND ITS DEVELOPMENT

PRO helps to associate the outcomes achieved with the care provided from the patient's perspective. Rising costs of health care and restricted funding environments have led surgeons to find cost-effective measures to sustain health care delivery for the present and future. Outcomes assessments with the aid of patient questionnaires can partially achieve this task. The federal government has devoted substantial funding for the Patient Reported Outcomes Measurement Information System (PROMIS) initiative under National Institutes of Health guidance in 1994. The primary goal of this multicenter (12 sites) research project is to develop valid, reliable, and standardized tools to assess PRO.[4] PROMIS uses item banks to generate instruments that can be used as primary or secondary end points in clinical studies that evaluate treatment effectiveness. These outcomes measures help assess various chronic conditions so outcomes can be comparable across studies.

TYPES OF AVAILABLE OUTCOMES QUESTIONNAIRES

PRO are obtained from patient interviews or questionnaires completed by patients during several follow-ups in the treatment process.[5] Two types of questionnaires are available for use: generic questionnaires and disease-specific questionnaires. Each questionnaire has certain advantages and disadvantages associated with them because they were originally designed for different purposes. As a result, it is important to differentiate between them before proceeding with their use.

Generic questionnaires are designed to assess the disease effect on the whole person irrespective of the medical condition. They are broad and can be used for an overall health assessment after an intervention, as an accompaniment to disease-specific questionnaires, and when disease-specific questionnaires are not yet designed and available. For instance, Short Form 36 (SF-36) and Sickness Impact Profile can be used in a variety of conditions. SF-36 is a widely used generic measure along with specific measures to assess eight health domains.[6] Generic measures incorporate various qualitative and quantitative aspects of human life.[7] Each questionnaire is unique, so they provide researchers an opportunity to work with one or few questionnaires simultaneously and an ability to compare outcome results across different conditions.[8] However, they lack the precision and sensitivity to detect specific changes after an intervention.

Disease-specific questionnaires are designed to assess interventions in patient populations identified by a particular disease. They are more responsive than general questionnaires because they are sensitive to detect changes due to focused questions. They are useful to evaluate specific interventions and differences between two similar treatments. For example, the Nasal Appearance and Function Evaluation Questionnaire can be used to assess functional and aesthetic outcomes after nasal reconstruction.[9] Similarly, the Carpal Tunnel Questionnaire is a valid and reliable tool to assess symptom and functional changes after carpal tunnel surgery.[10] The Michigan Hand Outcomes Questionnaire (MHQ) is another valid questionnaire with six health domains that is used all over the world to evaluate outcomes in patients with hand conditions.[11] It also collects the data on the unaffected hand to be used as a control for the comparison of outcomes.

A disease-specific instrument is designed to assess specific interventions. However, when a specific instrument addresses all aspects of intervention but fails to consider quality-of-life domains, such as psychosocial and sexual functioning, a generic instrument should be used as an accompaniment. For example, the Breast-related Symptoms Questionnaire used to evaluate outcomes after breast reduction assesses only breast symptoms.[12] A generic questionnaire can be used to evaluate a specific treatment when a disease-specific instrument is not available. For instance, Dolan and colleagues[13] used SF-36 to assess health-related quality-of-life outcomes after microvascular free flap reconstruction. However, the use of a specific questionnaire to assess general health cannot accomplish the expected purpose because it fails to incorporate the items beyond the specific condition. A list of available outcomes questionnaires in plastic surgery with their component scales and specific use is outlined in **Table 1**.

FACTORS AFFECTING THE SELECTION OF AN APPROPRIATE QUESTIONNAIRE

Most clinicians are not aware of the clinical usefulness of questionnaires to be used in their study, so user preference serves as a guide to choose the instrument.[7,14] Several factors, such as study sample, type of disease, and type of intervention, need to be taken into account when selecting a questionnaire.[5] The purpose of a questionnaire should be clearly defined before its use to assess outcomes in plastic surgery. Quality and content of the instruments are other factors considered important in the selection.[15] To evaluate the outcome of a specific treatment performed on a single patient at different points of time or on a group of patients, a disease-specific questionnaire is more applicable because it is more responsive to small changes with time. For example, the BREAST-Q can be used for outcomes after breast reconstruction in patients with breast cancer. To examine quality of care delivered and cost-effectiveness of interventions in different scenarios, a generic questionnaire is more applicable, such as the SF-36 or Sickness Impact Profile. To compare outcomes among different studies or to estimate the use of resources, a disease-specific or generic questionnaire can be used, respectively.[7] Overall, the purpose of research or the outcome of interest to surgeons or an outcome important to patients determines the choice of a generic or disease-specific (or sometimes both types) questionnaire in a given situation.[16] **Table 1** provides a list of outcomes instruments commonly used in plastic surgery.

STRATEGIES TO IDENTIFY AN IDEAL QUESTIONNAIRE

An ideal instrument yields accurate results in terms of demonstrating the true effect of an intervention.

An instrument that demonstrates good reliability, validity, and responsiveness to change is considered ideal to perform assessments. During the design and testing stages of an instrument, certain criteria must be fulfilled for an ideal instrument to possess these attributes. The criteria include item development, item reduction, scale development, field testing, and psychometric evaluation.[1] Previous instruments developed for similar conditions can be referred to guide the development of items and scales in a new instrument while adapting to the patient population and condition in context. Guidelines established by the Scientific Advisory Committee of the Medical Outcomes Trust and US Food and Drug Administration regarding criteria evaluation can be used in the instrument development.[17–19] It is therefore critical to ensure that the instrument selected for use in the study has incorporated these steps in the design process. This can be achieved by reviewing the literature regarding development of the questionnaire. Reliability of an instrument refers to the ability to produce similar results on repeat testing. Intraclass correlation coefficient measures this test-retest reliability; values greater than 0.9 are considered acceptable (range, 0.0–1).[20] Individual items within a domain or scale are expected to correlate with one another, referred to as "internal consistency reliability." The minimum standard for this reliability coefficient is greater than 0.7 as measured by Cronbach α (range, 0.0–1).[1,20]

Additionally, it is advantageous if the instrument possesses all the domains of the PRO it is intended to measure. This is referred to as "content validity," one of the two components of validity, which constitute the psychometric property of an instrument.[1] Involving patients in the item generation stage and field or pilot testing stage through interviews provides a stronger content validity than just referring to literature or expert opinion because these are PRO measurement tools.[21] Patient interviews help surgeons learn about the information most important to patients that may be overlooked by surgeons. The results obtained with the use of a new instrument should then be compared with an existing standard or other widely used similar instrument to assess its performance. This component is the construct validity of an instrument. Well-established construct validity adds to the value of a tool.

Responsiveness of an instrument is the ability to detect clinical changes in outcomes. In evaluating treatments, responsiveness refers to the ability to identify the changes from preoperative to postoperative follow-up periods. It is commonly expressed in terms of effect size and minimal clinically important difference of an instrument for that

Table 1
Available questionnaires for outcomes assessment in plastic surgery

Name	Purpose	Component Scales/Items	Developed by
Breast			
BREAST-Q[1,23]	To assess impact and effectiveness of breast surgery	Three modules: augmentation, reduction, and reconstruction. Six scales: psychosocial well-being, physical, and sexual well-being, satisfaction with breasts, satisfaction with outcome, and satisfaction with care	Pusic et al.
Breast Evaluation Questionnaire[28,29]	To assess patient satisfaction with breast attributes and quality of life outcome after breast surgery	55 items: degree of comfort with size, appearance of the breasts, and satisfaction level achieved	Anderson et al.
Outcomes of Plastic Surgery, hand/arm questionnaire[4]	To assess outcomes of plastic surgery of hand and arm	Symptoms, limitation of daily activities, psychological functioning/cosmetic appearance, and patient satisfaction	
European Organization for Research and Treatment of Cancer Quality of Life questionnaire C30[1]	Breast module (Br 23) items assess disease symptoms, side effects of treatment, body image, sexual functioning, and future perspectives	Nine scales: five functional, three symptom, and one global health-related quality-of-life scale. Used to assess patients with cancer	
Face			
FACE-Q[30]	To assess impact and effectiveness of facial aesthetic procedures	Four scales: satisfaction with facial appearance, health-related quality of life, negative sequelae, and satisfaction with process of care	Klassan et al.
Facial Injectables, Longevity, Late and Early Reactions and Satisfaction Questionnaire[31]	Physical and social experiences after treatment with injectable facial soft tissue fillers	43 items: patient demographics (4); patient satisfaction with treatment (10); procedure-related events (3–7); impact on relationships (9–15); and economic considerations (3–7)	Sclafani et al.
Facial Clinimetric Evaluation Scale[17]	Measures facial impairment and disability	15 items, six domains: facial movement, facial comfort, oral function, eye comfort, lacrimal control, and social function. Used to assess patients with facial paralysis	Baylor College of Medicine, Houston, Texas
Facial Disability Index[17]	Measures disability and social and emotional well-being of facial paralysis patients	10 items, two domains- social/wellbeing function and physical function	

(continued on next page)

Table 1
(continued)

Name	Purpose	Component Scales/Items	Developed by
Facial Lines Treatment Satisfaction[15]	To assess patient satisfaction with facial line treatment	14 items measuring facial line appearance, procedure satisfaction, and patient confidence	Allergan
Facial Lines Outcome Questionnaire[15]	To measure hyperfunctional facial lines of the upper face	Seven items	Allergan
Derriford Appearance Scale[1,24]	Physical and psychosocial aspects of facial and bodily appearance	Six measures of psychological distress and dysfunction and one measure of physical distress and dysfunction	
Rhinoplasty Outcomes Evaluation[15,27]	Used to assess patients after rhinoplasty surgery	Six items, three domains: appearance, functional outcome, and social acceptance	Alsaraff
Blepharoplasty Outcomes Evaluation[15,27]	Used to assess patients after blepharoplasty surgery	Three domains: appearance, functional outcome, and social acceptance	Alsaraff
Facelift Outcomes Evaluation[15,27]	Used to assess patients after facelift surgery	Three domains: appearance, functional outcome, and social acceptance	Alsaraff
Skin Rejuvenation Outcomes Evaluation[15,27]	Used to assess patients after skin resurfacing surgery	Three domains: appearance, functional outcome, and social acceptance	Alsaraff
Louisville Instrument For Transplantation[32]	Used to assess patients after composite tissue allotransplantation surgery	Quality of life improvement, aesthetic and functional outcomes	Cunningham et al.
Glasgow Benefit Inventory[15,33]	Measures general perception of well-being, social and physical well-being	18 items, general benefit scale, social support scale, and physical health status scale. Used to assess patients after head and neck surgery, especially functional and cosmetic rhinoplasty	
Aesthetic Surgery			
Multidimensional Body-States Relations Questionnaire[11,34]	To assess body image	Has psychological, body image, and general questions. 10 subscales to assess individual's satisfaction with five dimensions of body image	
Body Dysmorphic Disorder Questionnaire[25]	To assess body dysmorphic disorder	Four sets of questions	Phillips et al.
Dysmorphic Concern Questionnaire[25]	Used to assess patients with concern on physical appearance	Seven questions	Oosthuizen et al.

particular condition. In addition, responsiveness as determined by minimal clinically important difference helps in establishing the clinical significance of a study; if the study outcome scores are at or above the minimal clinically important difference, the study findings become clinically significant. As a result, evaluating the responsiveness indirectly determines the clinical usefulness of an instrument.

The reliability and validity of ad hoc questionnaires that are sometimes used cannot be ensured in evidence-based practice because they are not scientifically developed and psychometrically tested.[21,22] Readers can perform a literature search to identify the psychometric properties of an instrument that were established in the studies conducted earlier and thus select an instrument that possesses good attributes.

PEARLS

Although it is a laborious task to develop a questionnaire and establish its psychometric properties and at times practically difficult to incorporate its use into busy clinical practice, the use of outcome questionnaires endows plastic surgeons with several advantages. Scientifically devised and psychometrically tested instruments offer evidence-based results in response to the outcome assessments. Often plastic surgeons encounter situations when several treatment methods for a condition are associated with similar outcomes and similar complications, and literature fails to recommend a procedure. PRO through questionnaires guides surgeons to choose a treatment method with which patients are more satisfied in these circumstances.[1] They also help to evaluate different treatments, differentiate between various approaches, and potentially compare the results obtained by different surgeons in a systematic way.[2]

Outcome measurement tools can be used to perform a cost-effective analysis. Costs of health care are continually increasing, and to provide quality care without creating a huge burden on society, comparing the cost effectiveness of alternate procedures helps one to arrive at treatments that provide greater relief at less cost. For example, one of the most commonly performed procedures in plastic reconstructive surgery is breast reconstruction with different types of flaps: TRAM flap, DIEP flap, and latissmus dorsi flap. Using the BREAST-Q questionnaire to compare the outcomes achieved and cost incurred with the three types of flap helps identify the less expensive method to achieve quality reconstruction.

It is a good practice to administer the instruments that have been used in prior studies, or that have their development details elucidated in the articles. In the event of inability to find the conceptual background of a tool, reference into a study cited in the article for the development process of that specific tool can be done to obtain additional information. Each outcomes questionnaire is unique and distinct from others, thereby permitting the use of an additional questionnaire when one questionnaire does not seem to cover all the domains of treatment outcomes.

Overall, a PRO measure developed based on the guidelines allows the surgeon to compare techniques, quantify positive effects, and identify potential candidates for appropriate procedures from a group of patients.[15] It functions as a standard for future clinical trials. In addition, it helps the surgeon to have important patient feedback about the entire treatment experience that includes aspects beyond the procedure itself, such as patient education and communication before and after the procedure.[15]

PITFALLS

As an accompaniment to the numerous advantages of an outcomes questionnaire, surgeons need to be cautious about pitfalls encountered during their use. Most important is the selection of an instrument; an inappropriate tool used to make assessments will not be able to accomplish the purpose of its use. It is challenging to select a suitable measurement tool among the myriad of existing choices that pertain to the target population. However, the goal can be fulfilled if the choice is based on selecting a questionnaire that has been designed on conceptual framework and scientific background.

The use of instruments not specifically designed for certain types of populations does not yield meaningful results when they were not involved in the pilot testing stage.[2] For instance, the BREAST-Q is used to evaluate outcomes in women who have undergone breast reconstruction, but its use in women who have undergone lumpectomy or radiation may not be valid because these women were not represented in the initial design and development of the instrument.[23] It is important to ensure that the tools are used before, during, and after the intervention is performed so that the true effect is captured.[5] Specific attention should be made to the after treatment use because the time to follow-up differs based on the intervention and disease condition, and restricting to a time period that is too short may fail to measure the real outcome.

Poor design, incorrect use, and misinterpretation of scores lead to false inferences from a study; therefore, well-designed tools should be used according to the recommendations made by the developers of the instrument. Modification of questionnaires, such as adding or deleting items, rephrasing of questions, and translation to other languages, may affect validity, hence the psychometric properties of the modified questionnaire should be tested again with the new items before it can be used for the intended purpose.[5]

Use of multiple questionnaires or too many questions in one instrument may add burden on patients, reduce compliance, and require additional analysis.[7,8] Therefore, it is necessary to inquire if the disease-specific questionnaires are necessary for every plastic surgery condition or if similar results can be obtained from a more generalized questionnaire. For example, in a cohort of carpal tunnel syndrome patients, Kotsis and Chung used only two questionnaires, the MHQ and the DASH, and found that both questionnaires were responsive in measuring outcomes after carpal tunnel surgery.[8] Therefore, in future studies, use of either the MHQ or the DASH should provide sufficiently valid data to evaluate outcomes of carpal tunnel surgery.

The pediatric population, which may have different requirements with regards to item content and language, needs distinct consideration in choosing an appropriate outcomes tool.[24] The Derriford Appearance scale used for measuring the physical and psychosocial aspects of facial and bodily appearance is one such questionnaire that is not applicable to the pediatric patient. Likewise, SF-36 is a frequently used generic measure but cannot be used for patients younger than 14 years because it is not designed for that population.[6]

SUMMARY

The process of instrument development is complex and requires rigorous methods to ensure that the instrument possesses the necessary psychometric properties essential for the intended clinical purpose.[20] A systematic review by Pusic and colleagues[12] found that only 7 (3%) of the 223 PRO measures available in breast surgery were psychometrically tested for their use. They identified the necessity to develop reliable and valid measures in cosmetic and reconstructive breast surgery. Similar measures in other subspecialties of cosmetic surgery were found to be lacking.[15,25–27] Outcomes instruments that are systematically developed and validity tested need to be used in patients to assess surgical and nonsurgical interventions in a meaningful and responsive manner. Such an initiative will help to improve understanding of the effectiveness of interventions and quality of care delivered to patients.

The concept of using a psychometric scale in the form of questionnaires or surveys in routine clinical practice by a plastic surgeon is novel, but it is becoming standard practice because of its associated benefits. Increased use will help plastic surgeons to make appropriate patient selection for procedures and also to evaluate outcomes after treatment and for research.[24] Identifying the appropriate instruments that can be applied in clinical practice also helps surgeons make a comparison between studies and treatments. An example of a well-designed outcomes instrument in plastic surgery is the BREAST-Q, by Pusic and colleagues,[23] which adheres to the guidelines on outcomes instrument development.

If well-developed and validated tools are available for a condition, there is little need to develop new questionnaires except when they are simpler or provide enhanced information. In such an instance, the questionnaire needs to be developed in accordance with the scientific structure. The recent trend is to develop more region- or disease-specific tools because general questionnaires are too broad and imprecise for specific conditions. There should be a balance on how specific the questionnaires are developed. Instead, future efforts should focus on enabling the process of data collection and analysis through questionnaires simple enough to facilitate the regular use of these tools in clinical practice. Normative data need to be established for validated questionnaires to establish a reference when interpreting the scores from these tools. In the current era of outcomes assessment and evidence-based medicine, it is essential for plastic surgeons to be well-informed about the latest developments in understanding the assessment tools available to achieve enhanced patient satisfaction and quality of care.

REFERENCES

1. Davis Sears E, Chung KC. A guide to interpreting a study of patient-reported outcomes. Plast Reconstr Surg 2012;129(5):1200–7.
2. Alsarraf R. Outcomes instruments in facial plastic surgery. Facial Plast Surg 2002;18(2):77–86.
3. ASPS. Plastic surgery procedural statistics. 2012. Available at: http://www.plasticsurgery.org/news-and-resources/2011-statistics-.html. Accessed July 30, 2012.
4. PROMIS. Dynamic tools to measure health outcomes form the patient perspective. http://www.nihpromis.org/default. Accessed August 6, 2012.
5. Bindra RR, Dias JJ, Heras-Palau C, et al. Assessing outcome after hand surgery: the current state. J Hand Surg Br 2003;28(4):289–94.

6. Ware JE, Sherbourne CD. The MOS 36-item short-form health survey (SF-36). I. Conceptual framework and item selection. Med Care 1992;30:473–83.

7. Szabo RM. Outcomes assessment in hand surgery: when are they meaningful? J Hand Surg Am 2001; 26(6):993–1002.

8. Kotsis SV, Chung KC. Responsiveness of the Michigan Hand Outcomes Questionnaire and the Disabilities of the Arm, Shoulder and Hand questionnaire in carpal tunnel surgery. J Hand Surg Am 2005;30(1):81–6.

9. Moolenburgh SE, Mureau MA, Duivenvoorden HJ, et al. Validation of a questionnaire assessing patient's aesthetic and functional outcome after nasal reconstruction: the patient NAFEQ-score. J Plast Reconstr Aesthet Surg 2009;62(5):656–62.

10. Leite JC, Jerosch-Herold C, Song F. A systematic review of the psychometric properties of the Boston Carpal Tunnel Questionnaire. BMC Musculoskelet Disord 2006;7:78.

11. Chung KC, Pillsbury MS, Walters MR, et al. Reliability and validity testing of the Michigan Hand Outcomes Questionnaire. J Hand Surg Am 1998; 23(4):575–87.

12. Pusic AL, Chen CM, Cano S, et al. Measuring quality of life in cosmetic and reconstructive breast surgery: a systematic review of patient-reported outcomes instruments. Plast Reconstr Surg 2007;120(4):823–37 [discussion: 838–29].

13. Dolan RT, Butler JS, Murphy SM, et al. Health-related quality of life and functional outcomes following nerve transfers for traumatic upper brachial plexus injuries. J Hand Surg Eur Vol 2012;37(7):642–51.

14. McMillan CR, Binhammer PA. Which outcome measure is the best? Evaluating responsiveness of the disabilities of the arm, shoulder, and hand questionnaire, the Michigan Hand Questionnaire and the patient-specific functional scale following hand and wrist surgery. Hand (N Y) 2009;4(3):311–8.

15. Kosowski TR, McCarthy C, Reavey PL, et al. A systematic review of patient-reported outcome measures after facial cosmetic surgery and/or nonsurgical facial rejuvenation. Plast Reconstr Surg 2009;123(6):1819–27.

16. Wright JG. Outcomes research: what to measure. World J Surg 1999;23(12):1224–6.

17. Ho AL, Scott AM, Klassen AF, et al. Measuring quality of life and patient satisfaction in facial paralysis patients: a systematic review of patient-reported outcome measures. Plast Reconstr Surg 2012;130(1):91–9.

18. Assessing health status and quality-of-life instruments: attributes and review criteria. Qual Life Res 2002;11(3):193–205.

19. U.S. Department of Health and Human Services FDA Center for Drug Evaluation and Research, U.S. Department of Health and Human Services FDA Center for Biologics Evaluation and Research, U.S. Department of Health and Human Services FDA Center for Devices and Radiological Health. Guidance for industry: patient-reported outcome measures: use in medical product development to support labeling claims: draft guidance. Health Qual Life Outcomes 2006;4:79.

20. Alderman AK, Chung KC. Discussion. A systematic review of patient-reported outcome measures after facial cosmetic surgery and/or nonsurgical facial rejuvenation. Plast Reconstr Surg 2009;123(6): 1828–9.

21. Eckstein DA, Wu RL, Akinbiyi T, et al. Measuring quality of life in cleft lip and palate patients: currently available patient-reported outcomes measures. Plast Reconstr Surg 2011;128(5):518e–26e.

22. Pusic AL, Lemaine V, Klassen AF, et al. Patient-reported outcome measures in plastic surgery: use and interpretation in evidence-based medicine. Plast Reconstr Surg 2011;127(3):1361–7.

23. Pusic AL, Klassen AF, Scott AM, et al. Development of a new patient-reported outcome measure for breast surgery: the BREAST-Q. Plast Reconstr Surg 2009;124(2):345–53.

24. Harris DL, Carr AT. The Derriford Appearance Scale (DAS59): a new psychometric scale for the evaluation of patients with disfigurements and aesthetic problems of appearance. Br J Plast Surg 2001; 54(3):216–22.

25. Picavet V, Gabriels L, Jorissen M, et al. Screening tools for body dysmorphic disorder in a cosmetic surgery setting. Laryngoscope 2011;121(12): 2535–41.

26. Szpalski C, Weichman K, Sagebin F, et al. Need for standard outcome reporting systems in craniosynostosis. Neurosurg Focus 2011;31(2):E1.

27. Alsarraf R. Outcomes research in facial plastic surgery: a review and new directions. Aesthetic Plast Surg 2000;24(3):192–7.

28. Ridha H, Colville RJ, Vesely MJ. How happy are patients with their gynaecomastia reduction surgery? J Plast Reconstr Aesthet Surg 2009; 62(11):1473–8.

29. Anderson RC, Cunningham B, Tafesse E, et al. Validation of the breast evaluation questionnaire for use with breast surgery patients. Plast Reconstr Surg 2006;118(3):597–602.

30. Klassen AF, Cano SJ, Scott A, et al. Measuring patient-reported outcomes in facial aesthetic patients: development of the FACE-Q. Facial Plast Surg 2010;26(4):303–9.

31. Sclafani AP, Pizzi L, Jutkowitz E, et al. FILLERS-Q: an instrument for assessing patient experiences after treatment with facial injectable soft tissue fillers. Facial Plast Surg 2010;26(4):310–9.

32. Barker JH, Furr LA, McGuire S, et al. Patient expectations in facial transplantation. Ann Plast Surg 2008; 61(1):68–72.

33. Chauhan N, Warner J, Adamson PA. Adolescent rhinoplasty: challenges and psychosocial and clinical outcomes. Aesthetic Plast Surg 2010;34(4): 510–6.

34. Sarwer DB, Whitaker LA, Pertschuk MJ, et al. Body image concerns of reconstructive surgery patients: an underrecognized problem. Ann Plast Surg 1998;40(4):403–7.

How to Link Outcomes Data to Quality Initiatives in Plastic Surgery?

Jennifer F. Waljee, MD, MS*, Kevin C. Chung, MD, MS

KEYWORDS

- Quality of care • Health care policy • Patient safety

KEY POINTS

- The diversity of plastic surgery creates a unique and challenging opportunity to develop quality initiatives.
- Close attention to the principles of innovation dissemination can improve the adoption of quality initiatives.
- Innovative research with rigorous methodology is the cornerstone of developing quality initiatives that ensure patient safety and surgical quality.

OVERVIEW: THE EVOLUTION OF THE QUALITY OF CARE MOVEMENT

In recent decades, the accelerating cost of health care has sparked scrutiny of the quality of medical and surgical care delivered in the United States. For example, in the 1990s, evidence-based medicine (EBM) evolved to integrate clinical expertise, research evidence, and patient preferences to create the most appropriate evidence for clinical decision making.[1] In 1996, Sackett and colleagues[2] defined EBM as "the conscientious and judicious use of current best evidence from clinical care research in the management of individual patients." Furthermore, in 1999 and 2001, the Institute of Medicine published 2 landmark reports, "To Err is Human: Building a Safer Health System" and "Crossing the Quality Chiasm," which highlighted disparities in health care throughout the United States and the financial and societal implications of these variations.[3,4] These efforts underscored a national interest in using high-quality data to drive quality improvement efforts and create equal and accessible health care for all Americans.

Variation in health care may signal overuse, underuse, or misuse of health care resources, depending on the clinical context. Understanding the mechanisms that underlie variation has been the focus of a large proportion of health care policy and research.[5,6] For example, when scientific knowledge is unused or inadequately disseminated, variation may occur because of the inappropriate use of therapies and medical tests. Therefore, a quality initiative program can be designed to improve the process of delivering health care by using scientific evidence to identify and minimize variation, develop relevant benchmarks, and create strategies to achieve these

Disclosure: None of the authors has a financial interest to declare in relation to the content of this article. Supported in part by grants from the National Institute on Aging and National Institute of Arthritis and Musculoskeletal and Skin Diseases (R01 AR062066), from the National Institute of Arthritis and Musculoskeletal and Skin Diseases (2R01 AR047328-06), and a Midcareer Investigator Award in Patient-Oriented Research (K24 AR053120) (to Dr Kevin C. Chung).
Section of Plastic Surgery, Department of Surgery, The University of Michigan Health System, 2130 Taubman Center, SPC 5340, 1500 East Medical Center Drive, Ann Arbor, MI 48109-5340, USA
* Corresponding author.
E-mail address: filip@med.umich.edu

goals. Quality initiatives have been developed by federal and professional organizations to measure physician and hospital performance and adherence to recommended guidelines. For example, the US Centers for Medicare & Medicaid Services (CMS) collaborated with the Hospital Quality Alliance and the Joint Commission on Accreditation of Healthcare Organizations (JCAHO) to make measures of hospital performance publically available through the Hospital Compare program.[7] This program has resulted in improvement in patient outcomes, such as declines in mortality, hospital length of stay, and readmission rates. Therefore, developing effective quality initiative programs can measurably enhance the efficiency and quality of health care in the United States.

CREATING AND IMPLEMENTING QUALITY INITIATIVES

Although disparities and variations in care have been widely studied, the development and implementation of effective quality initiatives is challenging and often elusive. However, the process of information diffusion throughout a community has been well described in the social sciences, and the principles can be applied to health care. As outlined by Berwick[8] in 2003, the factors that influence dissemination can be categorized in the following way: perceptions of the initiative, characteristics of the community, and characteristics of the environment (**Table 1**).

Perception of the Initiative

For a quality initiative to be adopted, physicians, patients, and policy makers must have full understanding of the risks, benefits, and consequences of the initiative. For example, many aesthetic and reconstructive procedures can be safely performed in office-based ambulatory care facilities. However, in response to several patient deaths in office-based facilities, more stringent regulations were introduced by state and federal licensure committees to ensure patient safety.[9] Despite the increased cost and restrictions of these accreditation procedures, most outpatient plastic surgery procedures continue to be performed in office-based settings, and surgeons have recognized the need for more rigorous safety policies.[10–12] Quality initiatives must also be perceived as congruent with the needs of the population. For example, in 2011, the US Food and Drug Administration recognized the potential association between breast implants and anaplastic large cell lymphoma (ALCL) among patients who present with late periprosthetic seromas. In response to this concern, the American Society of Plastic Surgeons (ASPS) created a prospective registry of patients presenting with ALCL.[13,14] Given the vast number of women with breast implants for augmentation or reconstruction, this registry can define the natural history of periprosthetic seromas, elucidate risk factors for ALCL, and better inform women of the long-term risks

---

Table 1
Factors influencing the dissemination of innovation in a community

Factor	Involved Participants	Examples	Strategies
Perceptions	Clinicians Patients Policy makers Payers	Benefit Risk Costs Consequences (short and long term; positive and negative)	Education Transparent communication
Population	Initiative developers, leaders, executors, adopters of the initiative	Administrators, researchers, academic and community physicians	Foster early innovators, communicate with skeptics, facilitate uptake across most
Context	Leadership style Organizational structure and stability	Hierarchical structure Financial stability Ancillary support Patient population	Financial incentives Creating leadership roles within the organizational structure
Initiative	Compatibility Complexity Testability Observability	Community needs Simplicity of the initiative Ability to assess before and after effects Clarity of outcomes	Periodic efficiency and effectiveness checks Simple, easily implemented initiatives

of breast implants. In addition, the initiative must be perceived as simple and cost-effective. For example, in 2002, the ASPS launched a national clinical outcomes registry, Tracking Operations and Outcomes in Plastic Surgery (TOPS) in order for surgeons to submit sociodemographic, clinical, and outcomes data for benchmarking and evaluation. This dataset currently includes information for more than 500,000 cases and 1 million procedures, and allows surgeons readily to track and evaluate their patient outcomes.[15]

Characteristics of the Community

In addition to perception, the characteristics of the population that will implement the initiative influence its adoption. In 1943, a classic study of the rate of adoption of hybrid corn seed among Iowa farmers showed the principles of how innovation is incorporated throughout a community. This analysis revealed a sinusoidal diffusion of the use of hybrid seed corn among farmers over time.[8,16] Early adoption of hybrid corn is slow, and limited to a few farmers. However, a rapid phase of adoption then occurs, with a large number of farmers quickly changing their practice. The final phase is marked by most farmers using hybrid corn, and only a small minority failing to adopt it (**Fig. 1**). Each phase has characteristic features of the adopters. The innovators are the first to incorporate new changes, and are more tolerant of risk. In contrast, the laggards or skeptics are the last to introduce the initiative into their clinical practice, and tend to be more risk averse or traditionalists. In general, initiatives gain momentum and more widespread acceptance when approximately 15% to 20% of the initiative has been adopted. Therefore, the ability of innovators to initiate change within their environment is critical to initiate diffusion.[8]

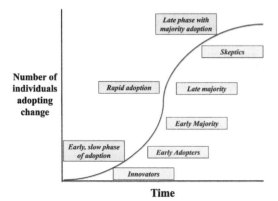

Fig. 1. The adoption of an initiation within a community over time.

Characteristics of the Environment

In addition to how the intervention is perceived and the characteristics of the adopters, environmental factors also influence the diffusion of initiatives. For example, the leadership and dynamics of the organization may be more or less favorable toward adopting new innovations. There may be external incentives readily available to those who adopt the initiative. For example, the use of information technology is higher among physicians who receive financial incentives compared with physicians who do not.[17]

Within this framework, several principles emerge for developing successful quality initiatives (**Fig. 2**). First, a successful quality initiative relies on sound, high-quality evidence that is relevant to the patient population of interest. In addition, strong

Define

Problem and current process

Opportunities for improvement

Potential benefits

Stakeholders and contributors

Measure

Current performance

Patterns and correlates of variation

Design

Intervention and evaluation strategy

Implement

Engage clinicians, patients, and administrators in initiative

Evaluate

Perception of initiative

Successes and failures of initiative

Patient outcomes following initiative

Educate

Inform future quality improvement efforts

Strategies to improve patient outcomes

Fig. 2. Steps to create a quality initiative in health care.

leadership by key stakeholders is needed to champion the initiative and spark interest and investment from the community. Furthermore, innovators are needed who will adopt the initiative early. Transparency and communication between policy makers and adopters can provide continuous feedback and optimization of the initiative. Examples of quality initiatives in plastic surgery are discussed later in this article.

USING EVIDENCE TO CHANGE PRACTICE: EXAMPLES IN PLASTIC SURGERY
Breast Reconstruction

Despite the psychosocial and functional benefits of breast reconstruction following mastectomy for breast cancer, rates of reconstruction in the United States are lower than expected.[18,19] However, the reasons for this discrepancy remain unclear, and may result from patient and surgeon factors, referral patterns, or social and financial barriers. For example, in 1997, a New York patient was denied coverage for breast reconstruction following mastectomy because the procedure was deemed cosmetic by her insurance company. In response to this, the Women's Health and Cancer Rights Act (WHCRA) was enacted in 1998, which mandated insurance coverage for postmastectomy breast reconstruction.[20] Although the patterns and rates of breast reconstruction have not changed substantially in the years following this legislation, this initiative has highlighted the influence of other factors that drive the decision for reconstruction, such as patient preference, patient knowledge, referral patterns, and access to specialty care.

Venous Thromboembolism

In August 2008, the Agency for Healthcare Research and Quality identified hospital-acquired venous thromboembolism (VTE) as the most common preventable cause of hospital death, specifically among patients who have recently undergone surgical procedures.[21] Although a significant body of research showed the effectiveness of VTE chemoprophylaxis among patients who have undergone orthopedic or general surgical procedures, adoption of such protocols remained sluggish among patients undergoing plastic and reconstructive surgical procedures. The reasons for this reluctance include concern for postoperative hematoma and lack of knowledge regarding the risk and effectiveness of chemoprophylaxis.[22–24] Therefore, in response to this concern, the Plastic Surgery Foundation sponsored the Venous Thromboembolism Prevention Study to examine the use of postoperative enoxaparin administered to patients admitted following

reconstructive procedures.[25,26] This effort successfully showed that enoxaparin effectively prevents the 60-day incidence of VTE among patients who have undergone reconstructive surgery without an increased risk of complications, specifically reoperative hematoma. With this evidence, investigators then developed a standardized protocol to identify appropriate patients for chemoprophylaxis at a large academic medical center.[26] At the initiation of the protocol, the adoption of chemoprophylaxis was 52% among surgeons; however, this increased to greater than 90% within 2 years and with sustained compliance. Professional organizations such as the ASPS are currently expanding educational programs and promoting the use of VTE protocols for patients having plastic surgery through Continuing Medical Education activities and prospective data collection to reduce the incidence of postoperative VTE.

Preoperative Verification

Despite conscientious and rigorous preparation, all surgeons are at risk of performing wrong-site surgery, including the wrong procedure, wrong patient, or wrong location. The National Quality Forum and The Joint Commission for Transforming Healthcare now consider wrong-site surgery as a never event, and numerous professional organizations have supported policies to perform preoperative verification processes to prevent the occurrence of these events.[27] Although wrong-site surgeries are exceedingly rare, root-cause analyses of these events reveals that, in most cases, no preoperative verification had been performed.[28,29] The Joint Commission has developed a standardized protocol involving all members of the surgical team, specifically nursing staff, surgeons, and anesthesiologists. This universal protocol includes a preprocedure verification process, preoperative site marking, and a final time-out before initiating the surgical procedure.[30,31] More recently, an expanded time-out has been proposed to encompass additional quality measures, such as preoperative β-blockade, antibiotic use, and intraoperative VTE prophylaxis.[32,33] Although the number of wrong-site surgeries that are prevented each year through these protocols is not known, preoperative verification procedures significantly improve collaboration and communication among clinicians, and contribute to a culture of patient safety in the operating room.[31,34]

Surgical-site Infections

Surgical-site infections (SSIs) are those that occur within 30 days of a surgical procedure or within

1 year of the implantation of a prosthetic device.[35] SSIs are the most common nosocomial infection, and are a significant cause of readmissions, morbidity, and mortality. Furthermore, up to 60% are potentially preventable with correct selection, timing, and dosage of perioperative antibiotics.[36,37] In 1994, the American College of Surgeons National Surgical Quality Improvement Program (NSQIP) was developed to compare observed and expected outcomes following surgical procedures to improve patient safety, with SSIs as a top priority for patient safety.[38,39] NSQIP is a well-validated, risk-adjusted, and peer-reviewed instrument that provides continuous feedback for the purpose of measuring outcomes and improving quality of care. Hospitals participating in NSQIP have experienced a significant improvement along quality measures with notable cost savings, and these were superior to other national quality initiatives.[40,41] For example, hospitals participating in NSQIP protocols have been shown to experience a 9% decline in the rate of SSIs.[42–45] Therefore, periodic feedback of comparative risk and outcomes provided by programs such as NSQIP can result in real-time quality assessment and improvement, ultimately yielding better patient outcomes.

CHALLENGES TO DEVELOPING QUALITY INITIATIVES IN PLASTIC SURGERY, AND FUTURE DIRECTIONS

Several unique aspects of plastic surgery create challenges for developing quality initiatives (**Table 2**). First, plastic surgery encompasses diverse disciplines, including craniofacial surgery, hand surgery, and aesthetic surgery, and many of the procedures performed by plastic surgeons overlap with other specialties. For example, orthopedic, plastic, and general surgeons may perform hand surgery procedures. The training and scope of practice for each of these surgeons can vary widely, and the surgeons are represented by different professional organizations. Therefore, it can be challenging to initiate policy changes in this diverse group. For example,

Table 2
Challenges in outcomes research in plastic and reconstructive surgeries, and potential strategies for improvement

Challenge	Example	Potential Strategies for Overcoming Barriers
Diverse specialties performing procedures	Rhinoplasty: otolaryngology, plastic surgery Hand surgery: plastic surgery, orthopedic surgery, general surgery Eyelid reconstruction: oculoplastic surgery, plastic surgery, otolaryngology Facial aesthetic surgery: plastic surgery, otolaryngology	Quality improvement initiatives developed by societies organized by disease and organ system, rather than specialty specific
Heterogeneous procedures	Breast reconstruction: autologous, implant based Reduction mammoplasty: pedicle design, skin resection design Rhytidectomy: deep plane, minimal access cranial suspension, subcutaneous	Tools designed to capture patient-centered outcomes (satisfaction, quality of life, aesthetic outcome, pain, return to work)
Rare diseases	Craniosynostosis Kienbock disease Poland syndrome Microtia	Multicenter prospective clinical registries that capture clinical end points and patient-centered outcomes
Lack of high-level evidence	Data supported by small case series or single-center studies without comparison groups	Adherence to the principles of EBM Multicenter collaboration to increase sample size Inclusion of comparison groups Randomization whenever possible

complex hand trauma is frequently referred to large tertiary care facilities because of a lack of available surgeons. However, rates of replantation remain similar, indicating that a significant proportion of these injuries could be managed without referral. Complex hand trauma reconstruction and replantation requires training and experience in microsurgical procedures.[46,47] Although the reasons for these referral patterns are multifactorial, many hand surgeons in practice may not have training in microsurgery and are reluctant to take on such cases.[48–54] However, establishing disease-specific professional organizations can unify diverse interests and facilitate the creation of quality initiatives, such as the appropriate referral for emergency hand care. For example, the American Society for Surgery of the Hand (ASSH) represents all surgeons who practice upper extremity surgery regardless of training background. This multidisciplinary society can reach a broader audience on relevant issues, such as hand transplantation, complex hand reconstruction, and Continuing Medical Education efforts, compared with specialty-specific organizations.

Furthermore, plastic and reconstructive procedures are technically demanding and highly dependent on surgeon experience and skill. Few procedures have a dogmatic, prescriptive approach, and there are a variety of procedures that can be performed for any single condition in plastic surgery. For example, for patients with breast cancer, multiple techniques for reconstruction exist. Although clinical and anatomic constraints guide the surgeon's choice of procedure, the choice of procedure often reflects surgeon experience and preference, and comparing long-term outcomes between different procedures can be difficult.[18,19,55] Patient-reported outcome measures, such as satisfaction, aesthetic result, and quality of life, can provide clinically relevant end points by which to compare procedures. For example, the Breast Q is a standardized assessment tool to measure patient-reported outcomes following breast surgery.[56–58] This instrument is sensitive to measure long-term satisfaction with appearance following autologous and autogenous breast reconstruction.[59] Other examples of instruments that provide standardized assessments of patient-reported outcomes following surgery include the Face Q following facial aesthetic surgery and the Michigan Hand Outcomes Questionnaire following hand surgery.[60–62] The data gleaned from these instruments can inform policy efforts, such as ensuring reimbursement for reconstructive procedures and the creation of patient decision aids.[20,63]

In addition to the heterogeneity of plastic surgery, many procedures are performed on rare conditions. For example, many congenital craniofacial disorders are exceedingly rare, and surgical procedures are typically concentrated among a few, high-volume surgeons in tertiary care centers.[64] Furthermore, the aesthetic sequelae of these conditions may take years to manifest. For example, cleft lip and palate repairs are performed in infancy childhood, but speech and aesthetic outcomes are not fully apparent for many years. To overcome these challenges, in 2001 the World Health Organization developed the International Database on Craniofacial Anomalies.[65] This registry collects prospective data from 62 registries and more than 2 million births per year to examine the risk factors and sequelae of these conditions. Therefore, establishing multicenter, prospective registries may allow clinicians to capture both clinical end points and patient-centered outcomes for rare diseases in an efficient and comprehensive manner.

In addition, one of the most significant challenges in plastic surgery is a lack of high-level scientific evidence on which to base initiatives.[66–68] It is difficult to create homogenous comparison groups that can be generalized to other centers, and it is often logistically and ethically challenging to randomize patients to treatments. For these reasons, outcomes research in plastic surgery has largely relied on small, retrospective case series, that are considered lesser levels of evidence compared with larger randomized controlled trials. Despite these challenges, important evidence can be gained from smaller studies while reconciling the limitations of the data.[69,70] Close attention to study biases, collaboration with other centers, (including comparison groups), and randomization whenever possible can overcome the limitations of the literature, and lay the foundation for future quality initiatives.

SUMMARY

Quality initiatives guided by strong evidence and championed by effective leaders can reach a wide audience and improve the health care delivered to patients. Although there are many examples in other fields of medicine, the diversity of plastic surgery disciplines often makes it challenging to develop quality initiatives. Nonetheless, close attention to the principles of dissemination of innovation and specific strategies to overcome these barriers in plastic surgery will facilitate the development of quality initiatives to improve care in this rich and diverse surgical specialty.

REFERENCES

1. Claridge JA, Fabian TC. History and development of evidence-based medicine. World J Surg 2005;29: 547–53.
2. Sackett DL, Rosenberg WM, Gray JA, et al. Evidence based medicine: what it is and what it isn't. BMJ 1996;312:71–2.
3. Institute of Medicine. Crossing the quality chasm: a new healthcare for the 21st century. Washington, DC: The National Academies Press; 2001.
4. Institute of Medicine. To err is human: building a safer health system. Washington, DC: The National Academies Press; 1999.
5. Wennberg JE. Time to tackle unwarranted variations in practice. BMJ 2011;342:687–90.
6. Wennberg JE. Understanding geographic variations in health care delivery. N Engl J Med 1999;340:52–3.
7. Lindenauer PK, Remus D, Roman S, et al. Public reporting and pay for performance in hospital quality improvement. N Engl J Med 2007;356:486–96.
8. Berwick DM. Disseminating innovations in health care. JAMA 2003;289:1969–75.
9. Clayman MA, Seagle BM. Office surgery safety: the myths and truths behind the Florida moratoria–six years of Florida data. Plast Reconstr Surg 2006; 118:777–85 [discussion: 786–7].
10. Haeck PC, Swanson JA, Iverson RE, et al. Evidence-based patient safety advisory: patient selection and procedures in ambulatory surgery. Plast Reconstr Surg 2009;124:6S–27S.
11. Byrd HS, Barton FE, Orenstein HH, et al. Safety and efficacy in an accredited outpatient plastic surgery facility: a review of 5316 consecutive cases. Plast Reconstr Surg 2003;112:636–41 [discussion: 642–6].
12. Rohrich RJ, White PF. Safety of outpatient surgery: is mandatory accreditation of outpatient surgery centers enough? Plast Reconstr Surg 2001;107: 189–92.
13. Bengtson B, Brody GS, Brown MH, et al. Managing late periprosthetic fluid collections (seroma) in patients with breast implants: a consensus panel recommendation and review of the literature. Plast Reconstr Surg 2011;128:1–7.
14. Eaves FF, Haeck P, Rohrich RJ. Breast implants and anaplastic large cell lymphoma (ALCL): using science to guide our patients and plastic surgeons worldwide. Plast Reconstr Surg 2011; 127(6):2501–3.
15. Alderman AK, Collins ED, Streu R, et al. Benchmarking outcomes in plastic surgery: national complication rates for abdominoplasty and breast augmentation. Plast Reconstr Surg 2009;124: 2127–33.
16. Ryan B, Gross NC. The diffusion of hybrid seed corn in two Iowa communities. Rural Sociol 1943;8:15–24.
17. Robinson JC, Casalino LP, Gillies RR, et al. Financial incentives, quality improvement programs, and the adoption of clinical information technology. Med Care 2009;47:411–7.
18. Alderman AK, Atisha D, Streu R, et al. Patterns and correlates of postmastectomy breast reconstruction by U.S. plastic surgeons: results from a national survey. Plast Reconstr Surg 2011;127:1796–803.
19. Alderman AK, Hawley ST, Waljee J, et al. Correlates of referral practices of general surgeons to plastic surgeons for mastectomy reconstruction. Cancer 2007;109:1715–20.
20. Alderman AK, Wei Y, Birkmeyer JD. Use of breast reconstruction after mastectomy following the Women's Health and Cancer Rights Act. JAMA 2006;295:387–8.
21. Maynard G, Stein K. Preventing hospital-acquired venous thromboembolism: a guide for effective quality improvement. Prepared by the Society of Hospital Medicine. Publication No. 08–0075.Agency for Healthcare Research and Quality. Rockville, MD: AHRQ; 2008.
22. Pannucci CJ, Oppenheimer AJ, Wilkins EG. Practice patterns in venous thromboembolism prophylaxis: a survey of 606 reconstructive breast surgeons. Ann Plast Surg 2010;64:732–7.
23. Pannucci CJ, Chang EY, Wilkins EG. Venous thromboembolic disease in autogenous breast reconstruction. Ann Plast Surg 2009;63:34–8.
24. Spring MA, Gutowski KA. Venous thromboembolism in plastic surgery patients: survey results of plastic surgeons. Aesthet Surg J 2006;26:522–9.
25. Pannucci CJ, Wachtman CF, Dreszer G, et al. The effect of postoperative enoxaparin on risk for reoperative hematoma. Plast Reconstr Surg 2012; 129:160–8.
26. Pannucci CJ, Jaber RM, Zumsteg JM, et al. Changing practice: implementation of a venous thromboembolism prophylaxis protocol at an academic medical center. Plast Reconstr Surg 2011;128:1085–92.
27. American College of Surgeons. The Joint Commission takes on wrong site surgery prevention. Bull Am Coll Surg 2011;96:70–1.
28. Kwaan MR, Studdert DM, Zinner MJ, et al. Incidence, patterns, and prevention of wrong-site surgery. Arch Surg 2006;141:353–7 [discussion: 7–8].
29. Stahel PF, Sabel AL, Victoroff MS, et al. Wrong-site and wrong-patient procedures in the universal protocol era: analysis of a prospective database of physician self-reported occurrences. Arch Surg 2010;145:978–84.
30. Clarke JR, Johnston J, Finley ED. Getting surgery right. Ann Surg 2007;246:395–403 [discussion: 403–5].
31. Michaels RK, Makary MA, Dahab Y, et al. Achieving the National Quality Forum's "Never Events": prevention of wrong site, wrong procedure, and wrong patient operations. Ann Surg 2007;245:526–32.

32. Altpeter T, Luckhardt K, Lewis JN, et al. Expanded surgical time out: a key to real-time data collection and quality improvement. J Am Coll Surg 2007; 204:527–32.

33. Hunter JG. Extend the universal protocol, not just the surgical time out. J Am Coll Surg 2007;205:e4–5.

34. Ring DC, Herndon JH, Meyer GS. Case records of the Massachusetts General Hospital: case 34-2010: a 65-year-old woman with an incorrect operation on the left hand. N Engl J Med 2010; 363:1950–7.

35. Trussler AP, Tabbal GN. Patient safety in plastic surgery. Plast Reconstr Surg 2012;130:470e–8e.

36. Hawn MT, Vick CC, Richman J, et al. Surgical site infection prevention: time to move beyond the surgical care improvement program. Ann Surg 2011;254:494–9 [discussion: 499–501].

37. Steinberg JP, Braun BI, Hellinger WC, et al. Timing of antimicrobial prophylaxis and the risk of surgical site infections: results from the trial to reduce antimicrobial prophylaxis errors. Ann Surg 2009; 250:10–6.

38. Khuri SF, Daley J, Henderson W, et al. The Department of Veterans Affairs' NSQIP: the first national, validated, outcome-based, risk-adjusted, and peer-controlled program for the measurement and enhancement of the quality of surgical care. National VA Surgical Quality Improvement Program. Ann Surg 1998;228:491–507.

39. Raval MV, Bentrem DJ, Eskandari MK, et al. The role of surgical champions in the American College of Surgeons National Surgical Quality Improvement Program–a national survey. J Surg Res 2011;166: e15–25.

40. Cima RR, Lackore KA, Nehring SA, et al. How best to measure surgical quality? Comparison of the Agency for Healthcare Research and Quality Patient Safety Indicators (AHRQ-PSI) and the American College of Surgeons National Surgical Quality Improvement Program (ACS-NSQIP) postoperative adverse events at a single institution. Surgery 2011;150:943–9.

41. Hollenbeak CS, Boltz MM, Wang L, et al. Cost-effectiveness of the National Surgical Quality Improvement Program. Ann Surg 2011;254:619–24.

42. Khuri SF, Henderson WG, Daley J, et al. Successful implementation of the Department of Veterans Affairs' national surgical quality improvement program in the private sector: the Patient Safety in Surgery study. Ann Surg 2008;248:329–36.

43. Guillamondegui OD, Gunter OL, Hines L, et al. Using the national surgical quality improvement program and the Tennessee Surgical Quality Collaborative to improve surgical outcomes. J Am Coll Surg 2012; 214:709–14 [discussion: 14–6].

44. Campbell DA Jr, Henderson WG, Englesbe MJ, et al. Surgical site infection prevention: the importance of operative duration and blood transfusion–results of the first American College of Surgeons-National Surgical Quality Improvement Program Best Practices Initiative. J Am Coll Surg 2008;207:810–20.

45. Berenguer CM, Ochsner MG Jr, Lord SA, et al. Improving surgical site infections: using National Surgical Quality Improvement Program data to institute Surgical Care Improvement Project protocols in improving surgical outcomes. J Am Coll Surg 2010; 210:737–41, 741–3.

46. Bueno RA Jr, Neumeister MW. Outcomes after mutilating hand injuries: review of the literature and recommendations for assessment. Hand Clin 2003; 19:193–204.

47. Neumeister MW, Brown RE. Mutilating hand injuries: principles and management. Hand Clin 2003; 19:1–15, v.

48. Sears ED, Larson B, Chung KC. A national survey of program director opinions of core competencies and structure of hand surgery fellowship training [abstract]. J Hand Surg Am 2012;37(10): 1971–1977.e7.

49. Ozer K, Kramer W, Gillani S, et al. Replantation versus revision of amputated fingers in patients air-transported to a level 1 trauma center. J Hand Surg Am 2010;35:936–40.

50. Chung KC, Kowalski CP, Walters MR. Finger replantation in the United States: rates and resource use from the 1996 Healthcare Cost and Utilization Project. J Hand Surg Am 2000;25:1038–42.

51. Chen MW, Narayan D. Economics of upper extremity replantation: national and local trends. Plast Reconstr Surg 2009;124:2003–11.

52. Mueller MA, Zaydfudim V, Sexton KW, et al. Lack of emergency hand surgery: discrepancy between elective and emergency hand care. Ann Plast Surg 2012;68:513–7.

53. Caffee H, Rudnick C. Access to hand surgery emergency care. Ann Plast Surg 2007;58:207–8.

54. Friedrich JB, Poppler LH, Mack CD, et al. Epidemiology of upper extremity replantation surgery in the United States. J Hand Surg Am 2011;36:1835–40.

55. Albornoz CR, Bach PB, Pusic AL, et al. The influence of sociodemographic factors and hospital characteristics on the method of breast reconstruction, including microsurgery: a U.S. population-based study. Plast Reconstr Surg 2012;129:1071–9.

56. Karanicolas PJ, Bickenbach K, Jayaraman S, et al. Measurement and interpretation of patient-reported outcomes in surgery: an opportunity for improvement. J Gastrointest Surg 2011;15:682–9.

57. Pusic AL, Klassen AF, Scott AM, et al. Development of a new patient-reported outcome measure for breast surgery: the BREAST-Q. Plast Reconstr Surg 2009;124:345–53.

58. Snell L, McCarthy C, Klassen A, et al. Clarifying the expectations of patients undergoing implant breast

reconstruction: a qualitative study. Plast Reconstr Surg 2010;126:1825–30.

59. Hu ES, Pusic AL, Waljee JF, et al. Patient-reported aesthetic satisfaction with breast reconstruction during the long-term survivorship period. Plast Reconstr Surg 2009;124:1–8.

60. Klassen AF, Cano SJ, Scott A, et al. Measuring patient-reported outcomes in facial aesthetic patients: development of the FACE-Q. Facial Plast Surg 2010;26:303–9.

61. Chung KC, Pillsbury MS, Walters MR, et al. Reliability and validity testing of the Michigan Hand Outcomes Questionnaire. J Hand Surg Am 1998;23:575–87.

62. Chung KC, Hamill JB, Walters MR, et al. The Michigan Hand Outcomes Questionnaire (MHQ): assessment of responsiveness to clinical change. Ann Plast Surg 1999;42:619–22.

63. Waljee JF, Rogers MA, Alderman AK. Decision aids and breast cancer: do they influence choice for surgery and knowledge of treatment options? J Clin Oncol 2007;25:1067–73.

64. White N, Warner RM, Noons P, et al. Changing referral patterns to a designated craniofacial centre over a four-year period. J Plast Reconstr Aesthet Surg 2010;63:921–5.

65. Mossey P. Epidemiology underpinning research in the aetiology of orofacial clefts. Orthod Craniofac Res 2007;10:114–20.

66. Momeni A, Becker A, Antes G, et al. Evidence-based plastic surgery: controlled trials in three plastic surgical journals (1990-2005). Ann Plast Surg 2008;61:221–5.

67. Chang EY, Pannucci CJ, Wilkins EG. Quality of clinical studies in aesthetic surgery journals: a 10-year review. Aesthet Surg J 2009;29:144–7 [discussion: 7–9].

68. Sinno H, Neel OF, Lutfy J, et al. Level of evidence in plastic surgery research. Plast Reconstr Surg 2011; 127:974–80.

69. Bhandari M, Guyatt GH, Swiontkowski MF. User's guide to the orthopaedic literature: how to use an article about a surgical therapy. J Bone Joint Surg Am 2001;83:916–26.

70. Bhandari M, Haynes RB. How to appraise the effectiveness of treatment. World J Surg 2005;29: 570–5.

Applying Economic Principles to Outcomes Analysis

Melissa J. Shauver, MPH[a], Kevin C. Chung, MD, MS[b],*

KEYWORDS

• Outcomes • Plastic surgery • Economic principles • Evidence-based medicine

KEY POINTS

• Economic outcomes are gaining stature as health care funding dwindles.
• The complex mix of payers in the specialty of plastic surgery makes collecting economic outcomes more difficult, but also more important.
• When creating or assessing an analysis including economic outcomes, it is essential that the perspective is clearly stated.
• To maintain a position of national policy relevance, plastic surgeons must include economic outcomes in analyses.
• In today's health care climate of scarce funding, it is prudent to include economic outcomes in comparative effective research whenever feasible.

In the 1950s and 1960s, as growing access to medical care led to concerns about increasing costs, research focus turned to the results of interventions.[1,2] This new attention toward the end effects of treatment was dubbed the "outcomes movement" and was labeled the "third revolution in health care" by then-editor of the *New England Journal of Medicine*, Arnold Relman.[1] Outcomes research strives to understand the results of interventions. These results are any patient experiences, including mortality, complications (or lack thereof), function, or quality of life, and can be reported by the provider, the patient, or by a third party.[3] As the movement spread, reporting of outcomes became almost cursory. The increased prominence of outcomes led to what some call the fourth revolution in health care, namely, evidence-based medicine.[4] Evidence-based medicine seeks to analyze and compare the outcomes, benefits, and risks of medical treatments, drugs, and devices to guide decision making by health care providers, consumers, and payers.[5] This is hoped to reduce rapidly growing health care spending thought to be caused, partially, by the lack of evidence for the effectiveness of many costly, innovative treatments.[6] Lack of evidence is not limited to new innovations, however; 85% of common medical treatments have not been rigorously validated.[7]

In today's health care marketplace, economic outcomes are increasingly becoming part of the assessment of medical interventions. Economic outcomes are indeed outcomes because they are a result of a care encounter,[8] although they are not typically considered as such. The rate at which new surgical techniques are introduced in plastic surgery makes the field especially conducive to the analysis of economic outcomes.[9] However, a systematic review of plastic surgery outcomes research from 1998 to 2004 found that only 3% of studies reported economic outcomes.[10] Possible reasons for this include

Disclosure: See last page of article.

[a] Section of Plastic Surgery, Department of Surgery, The University of Michigan Health System, 1500 East Medical Center Drive, Ann Arbor, MI 48109-0340, USA; [b] Section of Plastic Surgery, Department of Surgery, The University of Michigan Health System, 2130 Taubman Center, SPC 5340, 1500 East Medical Center Drive, Ann Arbor, MI 48109-0340, USA

* Corresponding author.

E-mail address: kecchung@umich.edu

Clin Plastic Surg 40 (2013) 281–285

http://dx.doi.org/10.1016/j.cps.2012.10.004

unfamiliarity of plastic surgery investigators with economic outcomes and that, for some procedures, costs are borne by patients.[9,11] To maintain a position of impact on health care policy, plastic surgeons need to include economic outcomes in their research whenever feasible.[10] The aim of this paper is to inform plastic surgeon investigators on the basics of economic outcomes and provide examples of their use in the plastic surgery literature.

WHAT ARE ECONOMIC OUTCOMES?

The most simple economic outcome is cost—the actual value of the resources consumed or depleted while providing a service.[11–13] Costs can be divided into several categories. Direct costs are generally the items one first thinks of when considering costs: Supplies, medication, and personnel.[11,13] Fixed direct costs are those that remain the same regardless of the number of times the service is provided.[11,13] These items, such as facilities, administrative costs, and durable equipment, cost roughly the same amount to own irrespective of frequency of use. Variable costs, likewise, are reliant on the number of times a service is provided. For instance, labor is largely dependent on the availability of work.[11,13] Combined with direct costs are indirect costs. These costs are more difficult to quantify and include items such as lost wages owing to time off of work or decreased work ability.[11,13] Even more difficult, or nearly impossible, to calculate are intangible costs, a monetary representation of non-financial outcomes such as pain, suffering, and even negative effects on relationships.[11,13] The final item in the calculation of total costs is opportunity costs. These costs represent the lost value when resources cannot be used in another manner. For instance, if an operating room is being used for a procedure that brings a hospital little income, it cannot be used for a more lucrative procedure.[14] This may be less of an issue for plastic surgery, because the specialty's hypothetical opportunity costs are low when compared with other surgical specialties.[14] To obtain a complete picture of costs, it is important to include all of these elements.

Costs are not the only economic outcome. Charges may also be the outcome of interest. Charges are how much is billed for a service, which may not reflect the actual cost.[12,13] Reimbursement, the amount received in exchange for a service, can be used as an outcome as well. In general, charges are higher than costs, owing to inclusion of profit and protection against uncompensated costs.[11–13] Reimbursements vary from $0 to the full amount charged and may be set by a third party, as in the case of Center for Medicare and Medicaid Services (CMS) reimbursement rates.[11] The tenuous relationship between these 3 economic outcome measures means that they are not interchangeable (**Fig. 1**). It is important to know which one is being used when a study is assessed. Likewise, when performing a study it is equally important to specify which outcome is being used.

WHOSE PERSPECTIVE?

When using traditional outcomes measures, it is easy for all parties to come to a consensus on what constitutes a good outcome. Patients, providers, and third-party payers can all agree that reduced pain is positive. However, matters of finances are less clear. Whereas patients may experience better aesthetic outcomes after a more expensive intervention, if the provider is not recouping costs, it is not universally favorable.[9] Therefore, it is important for researchers to be explicit about who is benefitting from the intervention under investigation.[9] This is important information for readers of published studies because only studies performed from the same perspective can be compared.[12]

The perspective taken depends on the research question being asked; there is no standard "best" perspective. Owing to the public nature of CMS reimbursement rates, assessing outcomes from a CMS perspective is relatively simple. Because other third-party payers base reimbursement rates on CMS rates, these figures can be extrapolated to third-party payers as a whole. With many plastic surgeons operating private practices, examining economic outcomes from the provider perspective can be enlightening, including specific outcomes, such as revenue (the amount earned) or profit (the amount earned after operating costs are subtracted). In the last decade, however, there has been a shift toward patient-rated outcomes;

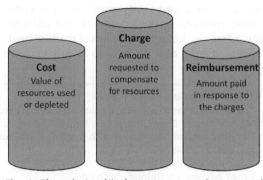

Fig. 1. The relationship between costs, charges, and reimbursements.

thus, there has been an increased interest in the economic ramifications of interventions on patients.[15] This is in line with movements to empower patients and encourage their active role in health care.[16] The patient perspective can be difficult to generalize. For procedures that are covered by third-party payers, patient costs can be negligible, placing more emphasis on indirect costs such as travel costs or lost wages, which are highly variable. The patient perspective is also the most likely of all perspectives to include intangible costs, which are nearly impossible to quantify. The societal perspective takes into account everyone who is impacted by an intervention, including individuals who are generally not considered, such as tax payers or coworkers who must work extra hours to cover for an ill employee.[12] However, including all of these viewpoints can be exceedingly difficult; to truly represent the perspective of society, members of the general public should provide values.[17]

Ideally, all costs that result from an encounter should be tallied, including cost savings if an intervention avoids a more expensive outcome, as well as difficult to calculate indirect, intangible, and opportunity costs[8]; however, it is impossible to include every item. For this reason, economic analyses are often based on a variety of assumptions, including estimated costs. Costs can be varied over a range of values to determine the robustness of the estimates to draw conclusions despite difficulty calculating exact costs.[12]

Examples in Plastic Surgery Literature

Provider perspective

When considering the provider perspective, whether individual surgeon, practice, or institutional, it is important to consider operating costs in addition to revenue. Given the perceived low reimbursement rates for postmastectomy breast reconstruction, Alderman and colleagues[18] sought to assess the impact of a variety of procedures on an academic plastic surgery practice and on the institution as a whole. Practice costs included physician salary, benefits, continuing medical education, malpractice insurance, and taxes, whereas institution costs were composed of fixed costs such as facility costs and variable costs such as nurse salaries and the costs of anesthesia. Also included were indirect costs, such as administrators' salaries. Revenue was in the form of reimbursements, and profit was calculated by subtracting costs from revenue. This analysis illustrates the importance of distinguishing between charges and reimbursements. For both the institution and the practice, reimbursements were

markedly less than charges. The institution received 56% of the amount billed, whereas the practice received only 32%. Despite this, overall an academic plastic surgery practice collects a profit of 27% for breast reconstruction, whereas the institution collects a 15% profit. To compare procedures, the authors calculated reimbursements by amount of time spent in the operating room. Delayed tissue expander plus implant reconstruction brought in the highest reimbursement/operating room hour, more than 5 times more than immediate transverse rectus abdominis myocutaneous flap reconstruction, which was reimbursed at the lowest rate.[18]

Alderman and colleagues[18] bring to light the issue of perspective, countering low physician and instruction reimbursement with evidence that patients prefer the aesthetic outcomes after transverse rectus abdominis myocutaneous flaps. Situations such as this are likely to only grow in number as our health care system attempts to balance financial constraints with an engaged public.

Third-party payer perspective versus patient perspective

Minimally invasive procedures may cost less, and may require less operating room time, often fewer staff, and generally shorter hospital stays. For these reasons, minimally invasive procedures are generally preferred by payers and patients alike. However, when hospital stays are shortened, there is often more home care involved and these costs may add up as well. Abbott and colleagues[19] compared the costs with third-party payers as well as non-covered patient costs associated with 2 treatments for sagittal synostosis: Cranial vault remodeling, which is more invasive and requires a long hospital stay, and endoscopically assisted suturectomy, which is associated with shorter hospital stays, but requires the use of an orthotic device and numerous outpatient visits. Third-party payer costs included both hospital and physician costs. Hospital costs included costs that could be directly attributed to patients, such as supplies and medication. Overhead costs, such as building maintenance and administration, that cannot be attributed to a single patient were included using a formula to estimate the proportion of these items used. Physician costs were calculated on a departmental basis by determining a cost-to-charge ratio for each specialty involved.[19] Non-covered patient costs were indirect costs incurred by patients (or in this case patients' families), including wages loss for hospitalization and follow-up visits, gas and auto wear and tear associated with driving to the hospital and to appointments. These are, of course, estimates based on patient populations as a whole; naturally, individually costs vary widely.

The authors found that cranial vault remodeling costs almost twice as much as endoscopically assisted suturectomy ($55,121 vs $23,377).[19] However, the costs to patients were significantly greater after endoscopically assisted suturectomy than after cranial vault remodeling ($3088 vs $2835, P<.001), owing primarily to cost associated with outpatient follow-up visits.[19] This highlights the importance of considering the costs to all parties involved. Treatment that is less costly to the health care system may increase costs to individuals. Although the cost difference to patients is minimal in this example, in some cases it may render the "cheaper" option unaffordable.

BEYOND ECONOMIC OUTCOMES: INCLUDING OTHER TYPES OF OUTCOMES

The practice of medicine is primarily about improving the lives of patients, not about saving money. Examples such as the previous one often lead to questions about more than costs: Which procedure has better outcomes? Which do patients and their families prefer? These questions require a more in-depth analysis combining economic and other types of outcomes. In such an analysis costs are considered along with outcomes to answer the question, "Are the outcomes worth the resources consumed?"[20]

Detailed instruction on the performance of an economic analysis has been published previously in this journal and is beyond the scope of our discussion.[9] Briefly, there are 4 broad categories of economic analyses: Cost minimization, cost effectiveness, cost utility, and cost benefit.[9,12] Unique to plastic surgery, outcomes tend more toward patient satisfaction or improved quality of life than toward mortality or life-years gained.[11] This makes cost–utility analyses ideal for the plastic surgery setting. Utility is the preference that one places on a particular health state, measured on a scale from 0 (death) – 1 (perfect health). Utilities can be elicited from a variety of populations, including patients, providers, and the general public, depending on the perspective sought. As with costs, it is important to remember that utilities can only be compared if they are obtained from the same perspective.[21–23] Utility values can be combined with the time spent in a health state to produce quality-adjusted life years, a method to place value on time spent in a disabled state.[20] This also allows the calculation of cost/quality-adjusted life years gained. Although the US government does not allow the

use of quality-adjusted life years to create payment thresholds,[24] a threshold of $50,000 to $150,000 is generally considered acceptable in most research settings.[25]

Example in Plastic Surgery Literature

Open fracture of the lower leg is a devastating injury. Amputation and salvage are the 2 treatment options and, regardless of which is pursued, recovery is long and often fraught with complications. Chung and colleagues[26] examined the 2-year and lifetime costs of amputation and salvage, as well as preference for these treatments. Costs were from the third-party payer perspective and included initial hospitalization, inpatient and outpatient rehabilitation, outpatient doctor visits, and the purchase and maintenance of prosthetics. To better estimate lifetime costs, dollar amounts were adjusted for inflation and for the discounted value of money over time.[26] Utility was elicited from reconstructive surgeons and physical medicine and rehabilitation physicians using an online survey.

Salvage was the less costly intervention both initially and over a patient's lifetime.[26] Salvage was also more preferred by providers, making it the dominant treatment option. Had amputation been the less costly intervention, further calculations involving QALYs could have determined if the cost savings were "worth it" in the opinion of providers. It is possible that the increased quality of life after salvage may be outweighed by the cost savings of using amputation.

BOTTOM LINE

Plastic surgery is a field that benefits from an influx of new innovations. Unfortunately, those innovations are frequently more expensive than those that came before them. This underscores the importance of incorporating economic outcomes in plastic surgery research as part of the best available evidence to support the adoption or rejection of interventions. This is complicated, however, by the matter of perspective. Whereas patients, providers, and third-party payers can see eye to eye on a number of issues, the inclusion of finances has a way of making matters thornier. The combination of economic outcomes with quality-of-life data can be an especially powerful tool for balancing competing priorities.[9]

Currently, many analyses focus on the physician perspective, either at the practice or institutional level. But as debate as to who is responsible to pay for health care (ie, private citizens vs the government) continues, interest will be drawn to the patient perspective and to the societal costs of interventions. The current health care climate is that of scarce funding. Although it is comforting to believe that health care exists in a vacuum where the cost of care and who is paying is not relevant, economic outcomes simply have to be in the conversation.

DISCLOSURE

Supported in part by grants from the National Institute on Aging and National Institute of Arthritis and Musculoskeletal and Skin Diseases (R01 AR062066) and from the National Institute of Arthritis and Musculoskeletal and Skin Diseases (2R01 AR047328-06) and a Midcareer Investigator Award in Patient-Oriented Research (K24 AR053120) (to Dr Kevin C. Chung).

REFERENCES

1. Relman AS. Assessment and accountability: the third revolution in medical care. N Engl J Med 1988;319:1220–2.
2. Chung KC, Burns PB, Davis Sears E. Outcomes research in hand surgery: where have we been and where should we go? J Hand Surg Am 2006; 31:1373–9.
3. Outcomes research fact sheet. Rockville (MD): Agency for Healthcare Research and Quality; 2000.
4. Chung KC, Ram AN. Evidence-based medicine: the fourth revolution in American medicine? Plast Reconstr Surg 2009;123:389–98.
5. What is comparative effectiveness research? Agency for Health Care Research and Quality; US Department of Health and Human Services. Available at: http://www.effectivehealthcare.ahrq.gov/index.cfm/what-is-comparative-effectiveness-research1/. Accessed March 21, 2012.
6. Pear R. U.S. to compare medical treatments. The New York Times. February 16, 2009; section A1:1.
7. Kocher MS, Henley MB. It is money that matters: decision analysis and cost-effectiveness analysis. Clin Orthop Relat Res 2003;413:106–16.
8. Khan JM. Understanding economic outcomes in critical care. Curr Opin Crit Care 2006;12:399–404.
9. Thoma A, Strumas N, Rockwell G, et al. The use of cost-effectiveness analysis in plastic surgery. Clin Plast Surg 2008;35:285–96.
10. Davis Sears E, Burns PB, Chung KC. The outcomes of outcome studies in plastic surgery: a systematic review of 17 years of plastic surgery research. Plast Reconstr Surg 2007;120:2059–65.
11. Kezirian EJ, Yueh B. Introduction of cost analysis in facial plastic surgery. Facial Plast Surg 2002;18: 95–9.
12. Kotsis SV, Chung KC. Fundamental principles of conducting a surgery economic analysis study. Plast Reconstr Surg 2010;125:727–35.
13. Chiba N, Gralnek IM, Moayyedi P, et al. A glossary of economic terms. Eur J Gastroenterol Hepatol 2004; 16:563–5.
14. Chatterjee A, Payette MJ, Demas CP, et al. Opportunity cost: a systematic application to surgery. Surgery 2009;146:18–22.
15. Bindra RR, Dias JJ, Heras-Palau C, et al. Assessing outcome after hand surgery: the current state. J Hand Surg Br 2003;28:289–94.
16. Alderman AK, Chung KC. Measuring outcomes in hand surgery. Clin Plast Surg 2008;35:239–50.
17. Wimo A. Clinical and economic outcomes - friend of foe? Int Psychogeriatr 2007;19:497–507.
18. Alderman AK, Storey AF, Nair NS, et al. Financial impact of breast reconstruction on an academic surgical practice. Plast Reconstr Surg 2009;123:1408–13.
19. Abbott MM, Rogers GF, Proctor MR, et al. Cost of treating sagittal synostosis in the first year of life. J Craniofac Surg 2012;23:88–93.
20. Drummond MF, Richardson WS, O'Brien BJ, et al. Users' guides to the medical literature. XIII. How to use an article on economic analysis of clinical practice. A. Are the results of the study valid? Evidence-Based Medicine Working Group. JAMA 1997;277: 1552–7.
21. Arnold D, Girling A, Stevens A, et al. Comparison of direct and indirect methods of estimating health state utilities for resource allocation: review and empirical analysis. BMJ 2009;339:b2688.
22. McLernon DJ, Dillon J, Donnan PT. Health-state utilities in liver disease: a systematic review. Med Decis Making 2008;28:582–92.
23. Mortimer D, Segal L. Comparing the incomparable? A systematic review of competing techniques for converting descriptive measures of health status into QALY-weights. Med Decis Making 2008;28: 66–89.
24. Patient Protection and Affordable Care Act. In: HR 3590–111th Congress. 2010.
25. Rudolph SH, Levine SR. Telestroke, QALYs, and current health care policy: the Heisenberg uncertainty principle. Neurology 2011;77:1584–5.
26. Chung KC, Saddawi-Konefka D, Haase SC, et al. A cost-utility analysis of amputation versus salvage for Gustilo type IIIB and IIIC open tibial fractures. Plast Reconstr Surg 2009;124:1965–73.

A Closer Look at the BREAST-Q©

Stefan J. Cano, PhD[a], Anne F. Klassen, DPhil, BA[b],
Amie M. Scott, MPH[c], Andrea L. Pusic, MD, MHS, FRCSC[c],*

KEYWORDS

- Patient-reported outcome instruments • Health-related quality of life • Breast cancer
- Psychometrics • Treatment outcome • Questionnaires • Outcome assessment (health care)
- Rasch measurement theory

KEY POINTS

- There is increasing demand for patient-reported outcome instruments in cosmetic and reconstructive breast surgery research and clinical practice.
- The BREAST-Q© consists of procedure-specific modules (ie, Augmentation, Reduction/Mastopexy, Mastectomy, Reconstruction) with independent scales that examine the issues that are most important to women who have undergone each procedure.
- The use of Rasch measurement methods to develop and test the scales of the BREAST-Q© means that there is a good understanding of the empirical item order across each scale, improving the ability to interpret the clinical meaning of scores as well as changes in scores.

OVERVIEW

In the past decade, our team has published extensively in the area of patient-reported outcome (PRO) research in plastic surgery.[1–8] The BREAST-Q© is the flagship of our research to date.[9–12] The motivation for developing the BREAST-Q© was that it is essential that surgeons play a central role in the development and application of PRO instruments, especially at a time when interpretation of such data is becoming vital to quality care.[8,13,14] PRO instrument development and validation is complex, involving robust data collection from large, heterogeneous patient cohorts, analyzed using state-of-the art psychometric methods. This article revisits the BREAST-Q© and expands on what sets it apart from other breast surgery PRO instruments.

WHY WAS THE BREAST-Q© DEVELOPED?

There is increasing demand for high-quality, specially designed questionnaires, known as PRO instruments, in cosmetic and reconstructive breast surgery research and clinical practice.[15,16] This demand is caused by the following factors:

- Outcomes data such as complications and photographic analyses alone are no longer

This paper is adapted from a podium presentation from the Joint International Measurement Confederation (IMEKO) TC1+ TC7 + TC13 Symposium *Intelligent Quality Measurement - Theory, Education and Training,* Jena, Germany, August, 2011.

Disclosure: The BREAST-Q© is jointly owned by Memorial Sloan-Kettering Cancer Center and the University of British Columbia. Drs Cano, Klassen, and Pusic are codevelopers of the BREAST-Q© and, as such, receive a share of any license revenues based on the inventor sharing policies of these two institutions. The BREAST-Q© is provided free of charge for academic research and individual clinical practice. The scoring software, Q-Score©, is also offered free of charge to all BREAST-Q© users. The BREAST-Q© is available at www.BREAST-Q.org.

[a] Clinical Neurology Research Group, Plymouth University Peninsula Schools of Medicine and Dentistry, Tamar Science Park, Plymouth PL6 8BX, UK; [b] Department of Pediatrics, 3N27, 1280 Main Street West, McMaster University, Hamilton L8S 4K1, ON, Canada; [c] Plastic and Reconstructive Surgery, Memorial Sloan-Kettering Cancer Center, Room MRI-1007, 1275 York Avenue, New York, NY 10065, USA
* Corresponding author.
E-mail address: pusica@mskcc.org

sufficient to support the progress being made in the field.[2]

- The public, health care payers, and policy-makers have become increasingly attuned to the importance of health-related quality of life (HR-QOL) and the patient's voice.[13,17]
- There is an emphasis on evidence-based practice[18] coupled with a new focus on key indicators such as HR-QOL and patient satisfaction.[2]

Despite the growing demand for PRO instruments, our systematic review found that none of the existing breast surgery–related measures captured a range of important outcomes in a scientifically sound manner.[15] Therefore, we identified a need for a new PRO instrument to measure the perceptions of patients having reconstructive and cosmetic breast surgery. In developing this instrument for cosmetic and reconstructive breast surgery (named the BREAST-Q©), we followed best practice guidelines.[13,19,20] Our methods, described in more detail elsewhere,[9,12,15] included in-depth patient and clinician interviews, literature review, focus groups, and cognitive debriefing.[9,15] We also strove to develop explicit descriptions of each scale, to maximize their usefulness as clinically interpretable tools. As such, the new PRO instrument was developed bottom-up (from a construct definition), rather than top-down (from a method of grouping items) to ensure that substantive clinically grounded hypotheses determined scale content. This process involved several rounds

of iterative qualitative enquiry using the methods described earlier to establish clinical validity. Our careful qualitative approach to content development is in keeping with the Rasch paradigm[21,22] (described later), and provided an optimal foundation to fully understand the measurement performance of each new scale.[23,24]

WHAT IS THE BREAST-Q©?

The BREAST-Q© is a PRO instrument designed to evaluate outcomes among women undergoing different types of breast surgery. There are currently 4 BREAST-Q© modules (ie, Augmentation, Reduction/Mastopexy, Mastectomy, Reconstruction), each of which comprises multiple scales. A fifth module (the BREAST-Q©: Breast Conserving Therapy module) is currently in development for women undergoing lumpectomy with and without radiation for the treatment of breast cancer.

The conceptual framework of the BREAST-Q© comprises the following 2 overarching themes (or domains): HR-QOL and patient satisfaction. Domain 1 (HR-QOL) comprises 3 subdomains: physical, psychosocial, and sexual well-being. Domain 2 (patient satisfaction) also comprises 3 subdomains: satisfaction with breasts, satisfaction with overall outcome, and satisfaction with care (**Fig. 1**). Body image, a key issue for breast surgery patients, is considered across multiple subdomains (psychosocial and sexual well-being, satisfaction with breasts). The 4 modules have the same conceptual framework, with the

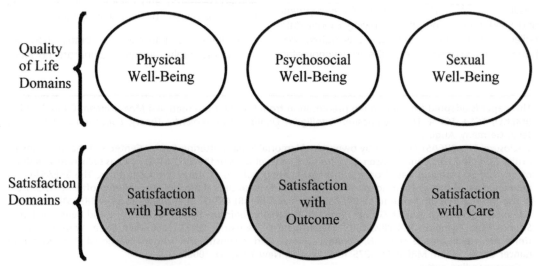

Fig. 1. BREAST-Q© conceptual framework. (*From* Pusic A, Klassen A, Scott A, et al. Development of a new patient-reported outcome measure for breast surgery: the BREAST-Q©. Plast Reconstr Surg 2009;124:345–53; with permission.)

exception of the Reconstruction module, which also includes the additional set of scales for measuring patient expectations.[25]

For each subtheme, 1 (or more) BREAST-Q© scale was developed to examine specific aspects of HR-QOL and patient satisfaction. For example, the Satisfaction with Care subdomain includes 4 separate scales that measure satisfaction with the following: information, the plastic surgeon, the medical team, and the office staff. Across the modules and patient treatment groups, the scales are psychometrically linked and can thus be used for comparison between different patient groups. **Box 1** shows the BREAST-Q© Reconstruction module as an example of the available scales.

Each BREAST-Q© scale is composed of a series of items (or questions) that evaluate a unidimensional construct. The items that form each scale reflect a clinically relevant hierarchy. As an example, in the Reconstruction module Satisfaction with Breasts scale, items span a range from "How satisfied are you with how you look in the mirror clothed?" to "How satisfied are you with how you look in the mirror unclothed?"

Each module of the BREAST-Q© has both preoperative and postoperative versions. The postoperative version includes all the preoperative items in addition to items that address unique postoperative issues (eg, scars). The preoperative and postoperative scales are linked psychometrically to measure change. Women may complete the preoperative questionnaire at any time before surgery (baseline assessment) and the postoperative questionnaire at any time point after surgery (follow-up data). The BREAST-Q© may also be administered at a single time point as in a cross-sectional survey. BREAST-Q© users may decide the time points to administer the scales. The BREAST-Q© Reconstruction module Patient Expectations scales differ in that they are designed for preoperative administration only.

Patients do not need to complete all BREAST-Q© scales in any given study or clinical encounter. Each scale is designed to function independently. Patients can thus be asked to complete some or all of a module's BREAST-Q© scales. A researcher or clinician may therefore select a subset of scales depending on the purpose of the particular study or use. As an example, in a quality improvement program, the 4 scales evaluating satisfaction with care might be used (Satisfaction with Information, Satisfaction with Surgeon, Satisfaction with Medical Team, Satisfaction with Office Staff), or the Satisfaction with Breast scale might be used alone in a study to evaluate a new breast surgery technique.

HOW IS THE BREAST-Q© SCORED?

For new PRO instruments to be appropriately used and widely accepted in different clinical scenarios, clinicians require well-targeted, reliable, and valid instruments that can also be easily scored. To achieve this requires both a psychometrically robust PRO instrument and a method of automatically scoring its data, based on items that are appropriately calibrated within a specifically defined, clinically meaningful, frame of reference. Scoring methods for PRO instruments have received little attention in the health arena.[18] Our team developed a stand-alone executable software application called Q-Score to allow data entry, automatic scoring, and export. The scores are generated based on scoring algorithms housed in the RUMM 2030 software program.[26]

Patient responses to items in each scale are transformed through the Q-Score scoring software (**Fig. 2**). Each scale has a unique scoring algorithm. The software provides the ability to read patient scale response data into the program, score the set of responses to each scale attempted, and write the complete set of transformed scores for all scales attempted to an electronic file. Once the set of responses are accepted, the program immediately scores these data and estimates a Rasch-based person measure, ranging from 0 to 100. This measure is based on the calibration of each set of items in each scale. All item response data, scoring, and measures can then be exported into a text file for further analyses.

There is no overall or total BREAST-Q© score, only scores for each independent scale. For all BREAST-Q© scales, a higher score means better HR-QOL or greater satisfaction (depending on the scale).

WHAT IS THE MEASUREMENT MODEL UNDERPINNING THE BREAST-Q©?

The extent to which a PRO instrument is interpretable and appropriate depends on the attention paid to the hierarchical clinical meaning of its content. The engine that operationalizes this content and drives the instrument is the measurement model that underpins the way the scales are scored. In health measurement research, there are 3 main psychometric approaches broadly based on the following 3 types of measurement model[27]:

1. Classical Test Theory (CTT)
2. Rasch Measurement Theory (RMT)
3. Item Response Theory

This article briefly examines the strengths and weaknesses of each approach in light of the

Box 1
BREAST-Q© Reconstruction module

HR-QOL domains

1. Psychosocial well-being. This scale measures psychosocial well-being with items that ask about body image (eg, accepting of body; attractive) and a woman's confidence in social settings. Other items cover emotional health and self-esteem.

2. Sexual well-being. This scale measures sexual well-being and body-image issues with items that ask about feelings of sexual attractiveness when clothed and unclothed and sexual confidence as it relates to the woman's breasts, as well as how comfortable or at ease a woman feels during sexual activity.

3. Physical well-being.

   a. Chest and upper body. This scale measures physical problems such as pain (eg, neck, back, shoulder, arm, rib) and problems in the breast area (eg, tightness, pulling, tenderness, pain). Other items ask about activity limitations and sleep problems caused by discomfort.

   b. Abdomen and trunk. This scale measures negative physical sequelae of the abdomen following autologous tissue reconstruction (TRAM or DIEP flap). Items cover abdominal discomfort, bloating, bulging, and pain as well as difficulty doing certain activities because of abdominal weakness.

Patient satisfaction domains

1. Satisfaction with breasts. This scale measures body image in terms of a woman's satisfaction with her breasts and asks questions regarding how comfortably bras fit, and how satisfied a woman is with her breast area both clothed and unclothed. Postoperative items ask about breast appearance (eg, size, symmetry, softness) and clothing issues (eg, how bras fit; being able to wear fitted clothes). There are also implant-specific items (eg, amount of rippling that can be seen or felt).

2. Satisfaction with nipples. This scale measures satisfaction with the appearance of the reconstructed nipple and areola complex. Items cover shape, color, projection, and how natural the reconstructed nipple looks.

3. Satisfaction with abdomen. This scale measures patient satisfaction with abdominal appearance following autologous tissue breast reconstruction (TRAM or DIEP flap). Items ask about overall appearance as well as position of navel (belly button) and scars.

4. Satisfaction with outcome. This scale measures a woman's overall appraisal of the outcome of her breast surgery. Items cover whether the woman's expectations were met with respect to the aesthetic outcome and the impact surgery has had on her life, as well as satisfaction with the decision to have surgery (eg, whether the woman would do it again).

5. Satisfaction with care

   a. Information. This scale measures satisfaction with information provided about breast reconstruction surgery from the surgeon. Items cover types of breast reconstruction, complications and risks, healing and recovery time, how the breast(s) would look, implications for future breast cancer screening, how the surgery would be done, and breast appearance (eg, breast size, scars).

   b. Surgeon. This scale measures satisfaction with the surgeon. Items ask about the surgeon's manner (eg, professional, reassuring, thorough, sensitive) and communication skills (eg, easy to talk to). Items also cover the extent to which the patient was involved in the decision making and understood the process.

   c. Medical team. This scale measures satisfaction with members of the medical team (other than the surgeon). Items ask whether the staff were professional, knowledgeable, and friendly, as well as how comfortable the woman was made to feel and whether she thought she was treated in a respectful manner.

   d. Office staff. This scale measures satisfaction with interactions with members of the office staff. Items ask whether staff were professional, knowledgeable, and friendly, as well as how comfortable the woman was made to feel and whether she thought she was treated in a respectful manner.

Patient expectations domains

These scales are designed to be administered preoperatively and assess patient expectations for the process and outcome of surgery. The expectations scales compliment the satisfaction and health-related quality of life domains of the Postoperative Reconstruction module. Multi-item and categorical scale structures are used.

1. Expectations for Support from Medical Staff. This scale measures how much time and emotional support the patient is expecting from the medical team and surgeon.

2. Expectations for Pain. This scale measures the magnitude of pain the patient is expecting to experience in the first week after reconstruction surgery.

3. Expectations for Coping. This scale measures how a patient is anticipating that she will cope with the process of breast reconstruction during the first year after surgery.

4. Expectations for Breast Appearance and Outcome. This scale measures how a patient expects her breasts to look 1 year after surgery.

5. Expectations for Psychosocial Well-being. This scale measures how a patient expects to feel about herself 1 year after breast reconstruction.

6. Expectations for Sexual Well-being. This scale measures how a patient expects she will feel sexually 1 year after breast reconstruction.

Abbreviations: DIEP, Deep Inferior Epigastric Perforator; TRAM, Transverse Rectus Abdominis Myocutaneous.

applicability of each model to the development of the BREAST-Q©.

CTT

CTT (or traditional test theory) was the cornerstone for psychometric evaluations during the last century in health measurement.[27] The key traditional psychometric properties commonly associated with CTT are data quality, scaling assumptions, targeting, reliability, validity, and responsiveness (described in more detail elsewhere[13,28]). These scale evaluations provide useful information about the measurement performance

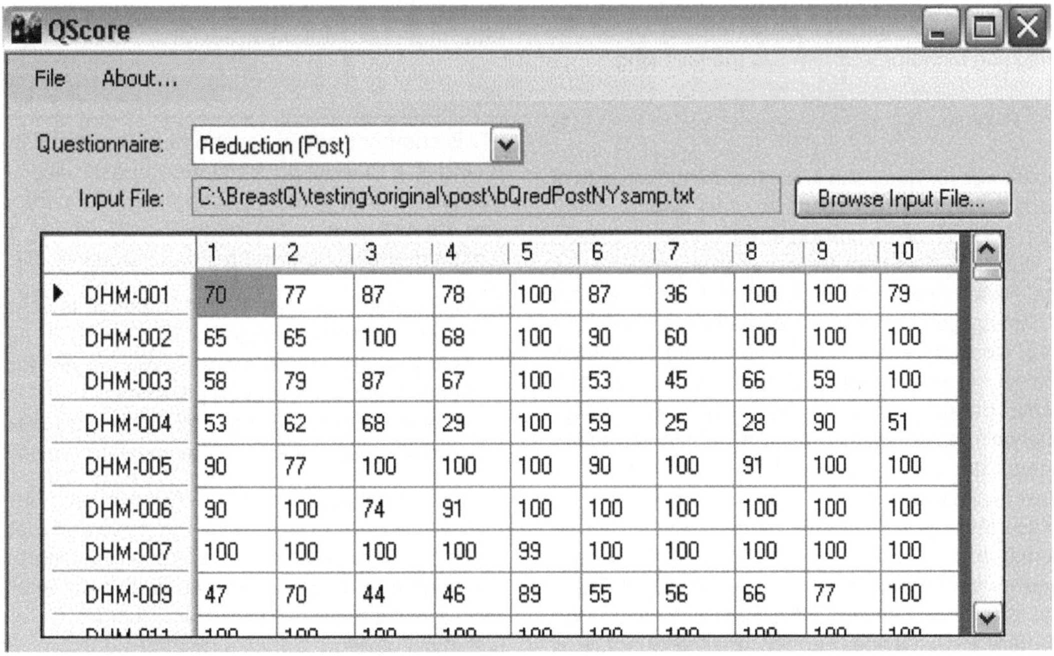

Fig. 2. Q-score user interface.

of PRO instruments. However, there are 4 main limitations of CTT. First, the measures generated are ordinal rather than interval (invariance is not hypothesized or experimentally tested).[29] Second, scores for persons and samples are scale dependent, because they lack a stochastic frame of reference, resulting in item parameters that must be regarded as fixed.[30] Third, scale properties, such as reliability and validity, are sample dependent. As such, the marginal probabilities of measures (ie, the probability distribution of scale scores) vary across population subgroups, because these subgroups may vary in the rate of the construct being measured.[31] Fourth, the data support group-level inferences but are not suitable for individual patient measurement.[32] Given these limitations, attention has now turned to newer psychometric methods such as Rasch Measurement Theory and Item Response Theory (IRT), which offer more robust psychometric measurement models.

RMT

Georg Rasch, a Danish mathematician, was principally concerned with the measurement of individuals rather than distribution of levels of a trait in a population. He argued that the core requirement of social measurement should be the same as that in physical measurement (ie, invariant comparison). With this in mind, he developed a simple logistic model (now known as the Rasch model). Through applications in education and psychology, he was able to show that his approach met the stringent criteria for measurement used in the physical sciences.[33] The formula for his model for scales including dichotomous items is the following:

$$\Pr\{x_{ni}|\beta_n, \delta_i\} = \frac{e^{x_{ni}(\beta_n-\delta_i)}}{1 + e^{(\beta_n-\delta_i)}} \quad (1)$$

where $x_{ni} \in [0, 1]$; β_n and δ_i are the measurements of person n and item i, respectively, on the same latent trait, and e is the natural logarithm constant (2.718).

Out of RMT is born Rasch analysis, which uses the Rasch model to evaluate the legitimacy of summing items to generate measurements, and their reliability and validity. The model articulates the set of requirements that must be met for rating scale data to generate internally valid, equal-interval measurements that are stable (invariant) across items and people.[29] The central tenet of Rasch analysis is that it examines the extent to which observed data (patients' responses to scale items) accord with (fit) predictions of those responses from a mathematical (Rasch) model. Thus, the difference between what should happen (expected) and what does happen (observed) indicates the extent to which measurement is achieved.

Statistical and graphical tests are used to evaluate the correspondence of data with the model. Certain tests are global, whereas others focus on specific observations, items, or persons. The following 7 key measurement properties should be considered: thresholds for item response options, item fit statistics, item locations, differential item functioning (DIF), correlations between standardized residuals, person separation index (PSI), and individual person change statistics. These properties are described in more detail elsewhere.[28]

Direct comparisons of CTT and RMT in the health measurement literature are sparse, and at best superficial.[34,35] In part, this may be because the 2 approaches cannot be compared easily, because they use different methods, produce different information, and apply different criteria for success and failure. However, RMT addresses each of the 4 limitations of CTT described earlier. First, the approach offers the ability to construct linear measurements from ordinal-level data, thereby addressing a major concern of using PRO instruments as outcome measures.[36,37] Second, RMT provides item estimates that are free from the sample distribution and person estimates that are free from the scale distribution, thus allowing for greater flexibility when different samples or test forms are used.[38] Third, the methods allow the use of subsets of items from each scale, rather than all items from the scale, without compromising the comparability of measures made using different sets of items, which is the foundation for item banking and computerized adaptive testing.[39] Fourth, RMT enables estimates suitable for individual person analyses rather than only for group comparison studies.[40,41]

IRT

IRT is another body of psychometric methods that provides a foundation for statistical estimation of parameters that represent the locations of persons and items on a latent continuum.[42] There are 3 main models under the general banner of IRT:

1. One-parameter (1P) model (identical in structure to the Rasch model)
2. Two-parameter (2P) model (includes an additional item discrimination parameter)[43]
3. Three-parameter (3P) model (adding a person guessing parameter[44] to the basic 2P model)[45]

The general approach in IRT focuses on mathematical models that explain the observed data. Thus, IRT scale evaluations are used to ascertain the degree to which given model and parameter estimates can account for the structure of, and statistical patterns within, a response dataset.[21,42] Models are postulated and examined relative to data. When the observed data are not adequately explained by the mathematical model (ie, when the data do not fit the chosen model closely enough), another model is tried. Thus, the justification for model selection is in the empirical evidence of its suitability.[46]

Justification for Model Choice

As outlined earlier, modern psychometric approaches, such as RMT, have substantial advantages compared with CTT for developing new PRO instruments. However, given the apparent similarity between RMT and IRT, does it matter which approach is used? RMT and IRT are mathematically similar, so they are often considered as members of the same family of statistical techniques.[21,47] Although they may be similar, the distinction between RMT and IRT has nevertheless important implications for clinicians and researchers.[21,47,48]

IRT models are statistical models used to explain data, and, as such, the aim of an IRT analysis is to find the statistical model that best explains the observed data.[21,47] When the observed data do not fit the chosen IRT model, another model is chosen that better explains the data. In contrast, RMT provides a mathematical model to guide the construction of stable linear measures from rating scale (eg, PRO instrument) data.[33] Therefore, the aim of RMT is to determine the extent to which observed rating scale data satisfy the measurement model. This tenet is central to the Rasch model and distinguishes it from IRT models. Its defining property is its mathematical embodiment of the principle of invariant comparison. These central tenets distinguish the RMT diagnostic paradigm from the IRT modeling paradigm.[21]

Therefore, in developing the new PRO instrument for cosmetic and reconstructive breast surgery, we selected RMT. In particular, we used the Rasch model for ordered response categories, which was developed for scales or tests containing polytomous items[23,49]:

$$Pr\{X_{ni} = x\} = \frac{\left[\exp\left(x(\beta_n - \delta_i) - \sum_{k=1}^{x} \tau_{ki}\right)\right]}{\sum_{x=0}^{m_i}\left[\exp\left(x(\beta_n - \delta_i) - \sum_{k=1}^{x} \tau_{ki}\right)\right]} \quad (2)$$

where $x \in [0, 1, 2, ..., m_i]$ is the integer response variable for person n with the ability β_n responding to item i with the difficulty δ_i and

$$\tau_{1i}, \tau_{2i}, ..., \tau_{mi}, \sum_{x=0}^{m} \tau_{xi} = 0 \quad (3)$$

are thresholds between $m_i + 1$ ordered categories where m_i is the maximum score of item i, $\tau \equiv 0$.[38]

This equation implies a single dimension with values β, δ, and τ located additively on the same scale. Thus, the set of positive integers x can contain a person's response to summated rating scales. For example, in the PRO instrument described in this article, the satisfaction-related items include response options containing the integers 1, 2, 3, and 4, which represent the semantic categories Very Dissatisfied Somewhat Dissatisfied, Somewhat Satisfied, and Very Satisfied.

The equation in the bottom half of Equation 2 is the normalizing factor, which specifies the probabilities of exceeding all thresholds for all categories preceding k, so that the probability of person n scoring in category k depends on all the locations of all the thresholds. This feature is important because it ensures that responses to items are constrained to a Guttman pattern, whose success is reflected by ordered thresholds. Thus, correctly ordered thresholds become an essential element of the validity of items,[38] an evaluation supported by readily available software[39] and theory.[40,41]

WHAT SETS THE BREAST-Q© APART FROM OTHER BREAST SURGERY PRO INSTRUMENTS?

The following 3 features set the BREAST-Q© apart from other related PRO instruments:

1. Focus on the patient voice
2. Strengths of using Rasch measurement methods
3. Practical benefits of an automatic scoring program

The Patient Voice

Overall, patient input proved to be the most important element of the content development process. In developing the conceptual framework for the BREAST-Q©, we sought to create a model that would reflect the entirety of the patient experience. Patients expressed both a sense of awareness of the impact of the procedure on their HR-QOL and an appraisal of the results of surgery (eg, satisfaction or dissatisfaction). The BREAST-Q© conceptual framework thus consists of both HR-QOL scales (Psychosocial, Physical, and Sexual Well-being) and satisfaction scales (Satisfaction with Breasts, Satisfaction with Overall Outcome, and Satisfaction with the Process of Care).

Patients in our interviews and focus groups repeatedly reflected on their relationship with the surgeon, the information that they received, and the care provided by the office staff. Process of care is measured by separate scales that examine satisfaction with preoperative information and the care provided by the plastic surgeon, the office staff, and other members of the medical team. These process measures may ultimately prove to be useful for quality improvement efforts. As an example, a plastic surgeon may use these scales to obtain useful metrics for individual practice improvement.

Benefits of Rasch Measurement Methods

The use of RMT to develop and test the scales of the BREAST-Q© means that there is a good understanding of the empirical item order across each scale. Thus, the items that are associated with every possible scale score are known. For example, using the BREAST-Q© Reconstruction Satisfaction with Breasts scale (described earlier), a multicenter, cross-sectional study of 672 post-mastectomy women, conducted by our group, found that women's satisfaction with their breasts was significantly greater among those who received silicone implants compared with those who received saline implants.[6] To interpret the scores further, the items in the range of the scale scores for the silicone group (mean score 64) and the saline group (mean score 57; **Fig. 3**) can be examined.

These scores translate into the following: women in the silicone group scored higher up the scale and, therefore, were typically satisfied with the look and feel of their reconstructed breasts, whereas women in the saline group scored more toward the middle of the scale and were satisfied with size and look of their breasts, but not how well they match or whether they feel natural. The ability to provide qualitative statements to scores for each group on each scale begins to verify the meaning of scale scores and thus provides a clear base for the clinical interpretation of the BREAST-Q©.[8]

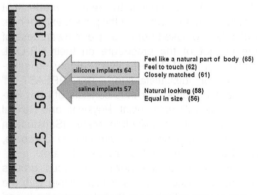

Fig. 3. Comparison of saline group and silicone group mean scores on the ruler of BREAST-Q© reconstruction scale of satisfaction with breasts.

A Practical Solution to Scoring

PRO instrument users have traditionally been required to handle data manually, producing total scores via scoring syntax in statistical software packages or other similar tools. These requirements can be a barrier to the use of PRO instruments, especially for clinicians in busy practices or clinical researchers who are using these instruments as part of a larger study. Overcoming these barriers is especially relevant in the context of the more complex algorithms and software associated with RMT. The new Q-Score© program offers a ready solution to this issue because it provides an easy, automatic, convenient, and tangible 0 to 100 score transformation that maintains a common frame of reference and metric comparability across different clinical samples. Scores, which are linearized (not ordinal) measures, satisfy statistical assumptions of unit additivity and support both group and individual patient-level comparisons.

WHAT IS NEXT FOR THE BREAST-Q©?

As an increasing number of researchers and surgeons incorporate the BREAST-Q© into their studies and surgical practices, we envision a rapidly expanding knowledge base that will inform further clinical interpretation of BREAST-Q© data. Thus, as BREAST-Q© data are collected in different clinical scenarios, the interpretation and the clinical meaning of scale scores will become increasingly clear. To optimally manage surgical patients in an increasingly cost-restricted environment, the BREAST-Q© can be used to provide meaningful data to guide the development of new techniques and devices, regulatory efforts, determination of comparative effectiveness, and patient advocacy.

REFERENCES

1. Fitzpatrick R, Jenkinson C, Klassen A, et al. Methods of assessing health-related quality of life and outcome for plastic surgery. Br J Plast Surg 1999;52:251–5.
2. Cano S, Browne J, Lamping D. Patient-based measures of outcome in plastic surgery: current approaches and future directions. Br J Plast Surg 2004;57:1–11.
3. Cano S, Klassen A, Pusic A. The science behind quality-of-life measurement: a primer for plastic surgeons. Plast Reconstr Surg 2009;123:98e–106e.
4. Kosowski T, McCarthy C, Reavey P, et al. A systematic review of patient-reported outcome measures after facial cosmetic surgery and/or nonsurgical facial rejuvenation. Plast Reconstr Surg 2009;123:1819–27.
5. Chen C, Cano S, Klassen A, et al. Measuring quality of life in oncologic breast surgery: a systematic review

of patient-reported outcome measures. Breast J 2010;16:587–97.

6. McCarthy C, Klassen A, Cano S, et al. Patient satisfaction with postmastectomy breast reconstruction: a comparison of saline and silicone implants. Cancer 2010;116:5584–91.

7. Reavey P, Klassen A, Cano S, et al. Measuring quality of life and patient satisfaction after body contouring: a systematic review of patient-reported outcome measures. Aesthet Surg J 2011;31:807–13.

8. Cano S, Klassen A, Scott A, et al. Health outcome and economic measurement in breast cancer surgery: challenges and opportunities. Expert Rev Pharmacoecon Outcomes Res 2010;10:583–94.

9. Klassen A, Pusic A, Scott A, et al. Satisfaction and quality of life in women who undergo breast surgery: a qualitative study. BMC Womens Health 2009;9:11–8.

10. Pusic A, McCarthy C, Cano S, et al. Clinical research in breast surgery: reduction and postmastectomy reconstruction. Clin Plast Surg 2008;35:215–26.

11. Pusic A, Reavey P, Klassen A, et al. Measuring patient outcomes in breast augmentation: introducing the BREAST-Q augmentation module. Clin Plast Surg 2009;36:23–32, v.

12. Cano S, Klassen A, Scott A, et al. The BREAST-Q ©: further validation in independent clinical samples. Plast Reconstr Surg 2012;129:293–302.

13. Food and Drug Administration. Patient reported outcome measures: use in medical product development to support labelling claims. Food and Drug Administration 2009.

14. Ahmed S, Berzon R, Revicki D, et al. The use of patient-reported outcomes (PRO) within comparative effectiveness research: implications for clinical practice and health care policy. Med Care 2012; 50(12):1060–70.

15. Pusic A, Klassen A, Scott A, et al. Development of a new patient-reported outcome measure for breast surgery: the BREAST-Q. Plast Reconstr Surg 2009; 124:345–53.

16. Pusic A, Chen CM, Cano S, et al. Measuring quality of life in cosmetic and reconstructive breast surgery: a systematic review of patient-reported outcomes instruments. Plast Reconstr Surg 2007;120:823–37 [discussion: 838–9].

17. UK Department of Health. Equity and excellence: liberating the NHS. London: Her Majesty's Stationery Office; 2010.

18. Institute of Medicine and National Research Council. Crossing the quality chasm: the IOM health care quality initiative. Washington, DC: The National Academies Press; 2001.

19. Scientific Advisory Committee of the Medical Outcomes Trust. Assessing health status and quality of life instruments: attributes and review criteria. Qual Life Res 2002;11:193–205.

20. Revicki D. FDA draft guidance and health-outcomes research. Lancet 2007;369:540–2.

21. Andrich D. Controversy and the Rasch model: a characteristic of incompatible paradigms? Med Care 2004;42:17–116.

22. Wilson M. Constructing measures: an item response modelling approach. Mahwah (NJ): Lawrence Erlbaum Associates; 2005.

23. Andrich D, de Jong J, Sheridan B. Diagnostic opportunities with the Rasch model for ordered response categories. In: Rost J, Langeheine R, editors. Applications of latent trait and latent class models in the social sciences. Munster (Germany): Waxmann Verlag; 1997. p. 59–70.

24. Fisher W, Stenner A. Integrating qualitative and quantitative research approaches via the phenomenological method. Int J Mult Res Approaches 2011; 5:89–103.

25. Snell L, McCarthy C, Klassen A, et al. Clarifying the expectations of patients undergoing implant breast reconstruction: a qualitative study. Plast Reconstr Surg 2010;126:1825–30.

26. Andrich D, Sheridan B. RUMM 2030. Perth (WA): RUMM Laboratory; 1997–2012.

27. Cano S, Hobart J. The problem with health measurement. Patient Prefer Adherence 2011;5: 279–90.

28. Hobart J, Cano S. Improving the evaluation of therapeutic intervention in MS: the role of new psychometric methods. Health Technol Assess 2009;13:1–200.

29. Wright B, Linacre J. Observations are always ordinal: measurements, however, must be interval. Arch Phys Med Rehabil 1989;70:857–60.

30. Embretson S, Hershberger S, editors. The new rules of measurement. Mahwah (NJ): Lawrence Erlbaum Associates; 1999.

31. Cano S, Posner H, Moline M, et al. The ADAS-cog in Alzheimer's disease clinical trials: psychometric evaluation of the sum and its parts. J Neurol Neurosurg Psychiatry 2010;81:1363–8.

32. McHorney C, Tarlov A. Individual-patient monitoring in clinical practice: are available health status surveys adequate? Qual Life Res 1995;4:293–307.

33. Rasch G. Probabilistic models for some intelligence and attainment tests. Copenhagen: Danish Institute for Education Research. 1960.

34. McHorney C, Haley S, Ware JJ. Evaluation of the MOS SF-36 Physical Functioning Scale (PF-10): II. Comparison of relative precision using Likert and Rasch scoring methods. J Clin Epidemiol 1997;50:451–61.

35. Prieto L, Alonso J, Lamarca R. Classical test theory versus Rasch analysis for quality of life questionnaire reduction. Health Qual Life Outcomes 2003; 1:27.

36. Whitaker J, McFarland H, Rudge P, et al. Outcomes assessment in multiple sclerosis trials: a critical analysis. Mult Scler 1995;1:37–47.

37. Platz T, Eickhof C, Nuyens G, et al. Clinical scales for the assessment of spasticity, associated phenomena, and function: a systematic review of the literature. Disabil Rehabil 2005;27:7–18.

38. Wright B, Masters G. Rating scale analysis: Rasch measurement. Chicago: MESA; 1982.

39. Linacre J. Computer-adaptive testing: a methodology whose time has come. In: Chae S, Kang U, Jeon E, et al, editors. Development of computerised middle school achievement tests. Seoul (South Korea): Komesa Press; 2000. p. 1–58.

40. Wright BD. Solving measurement problems with the Rasch model. J Educ Meas 1977;14:97–116.

41. Andrich D. Rasch models for measurement. Beverley Hills (CA): Sage Publications; 1988.

42. Lord F, Novick M. Statistical theories of mental test scores. Reading (MA): Addison-Wesley; 1968.

43. Lumsden J. Person reliability. Appl Psychol Meas 1977;1:477–82.

44. Waller M. Estimating parameters in the Rasch model: removing the effects of random guessing. Princeton (NJ): Educational Testing service; 1976.

45. Birnbaum A. Some latent trait models and their use in inferring an examinee's ability. In: Lord FM, Novick MR, editors. Statistical theories of mental test scores. Reading (MA): Addison-Wesley; 1968. p. 397–422.

46. Novick M. The axioms and principal results of classical test theory. J Math Psychol 1966;3:1–18.

47. Massof R. The measurement of vision disability. Optom Vis Sci 2002;79:516–52.

48. Hobart J, Cano S, Zajicek J, et al. Rating scales as outcome measures for clinical trials in neurology: problems, solutions, and recommendations. Lancet Neurol 2007;6:1094–105.

49. Andrich D. A rating formulation for ordered response categories. Psychometrika 1978;43:561–73.

Measuring Outcomes in Aesthetic Surgery

Amy Alderman, MD, MPH[a],*, Kevin C. Chung, MD, MS[b]

KEYWORDS

- Evidence-based medicine • Outcomes • Plastic surgery • Conceptual models • Decision-making

KEY POINTS

- The assessment of aesthetic surgery outcomes still has the basic, yet fundamental, question to answer: whose perspective on outcomes—the patient's or the physician's—is of primary importance?
- Because scientific data are difficult to distill from the aesthetic literature, significant challenges exist to integrate evidence-based medicine principles into the art of aesthetic surgery.
- Aesthetic surgery is an unusual doctor-patient relationship in which the patient is the sole consumer of elective services with no third-party payer involvement.
- The traditional balance of power between the physician and patient shifts toward the patient in elective procedures, elevating the importance of patient satisfaction with the surgical outcome.
- Evidence-based research is absolutely necessary to ensure high-quality care, and better study designs and measures will help create clinically meaningful outcomes.

INTRODUCTION

Evidence-based medicine (EBM) is being embraced by plastic surgery. Patient values are combined with scientific data to complement a plastic surgeon's clinical experience.[1] Aesthetic surgeons have also supported the EBM movement by attending the EBM summit convened by plastic surgery leadership in Colorado Springs in 2010. However, because scientific data are difficult to distill from the aesthetic literature, there are significant challenges to integrating EBM principles into the art of aesthetic surgery.[2] The primary dilemmas are to define the desired goals of aesthetic surgery and determine how outcomes can be measured; these challenges still face this subspecialty of plastic surgery.

Aesthetic surgery outcomes can be grouped into two primary domains: (1) complications and revisional surgery and (2) satisfaction with aesthetic outcomes.

Similar to other surgical fields, complications are well-defined, but revisional surgery rates can be variable depending on a surgeon's and a patient's willingness and desire for revisional surgery. Measuring satisfaction, however, is much more complex. Whose perspective takes primary importance—the patient or the surgeon? If the surgeon is satisfied with the aesthetic results, but the patient is not, is that a good outcome? What if the patient, not the surgeon, believes the outcome is good? Furthermore, patients' and surgeons' concept of beauty will vary dramatically across

Disclosure: Supported in part by grants from the National Institute on Aging, National Institute of Arthritis and Musculoskeletal and Skin Diseases (R01 AR062066), and the National Institute of Arthritis and Musculoskeletal and Skin Diseases (2R01 AR047328-06); and a Midcareer Investigator Award in Patient-Oriented Research (K24 AR053120) (to Dr Kevin C. Chung).
a Private practice, Atlanta, GA, USA; b Section of Plastic Surgery, The University of Michigan Medical School, MI, USA
* Corresponding author. Swan Center for Plastic Surgery, 4165 Old Milton Parkway, Suite 200 East, Alpharetta, GA 30005.
E-mail address: amyaldermanmd@yahoo.com

Clin Plastic Surg 40 (2013) 297–304
http://dx.doi.org/10.1016/j.cps.2012.10.005
0094-1298/13/$ – see front matter © 2013 Elsevier Inc. All rights reserved.

racial and/or ethnic backgrounds, geographic regions, and socioeconomic status.

CONCEPTUAL FRAMEWORK

When assessing any surgical outcome, whether aesthetic or reconstructive in nature, a conceptual framework should guide the research. The conceptual framework is a process-of-care roadmap that incorporates patient and external factors that can influence surgical outcomes. Examples of conceptual frameworks that could be used to assess aesthetic surgery outcomes are the Transtheoretical Model, Stages of Change Construct, and the Health Belief Model.[3] The Transtheoretical Model and Stages of Change Construct propose that patients move through a series of steps or stages when making decisions and taking actions about their health and the health care they receive. The stages are defined by their differing degrees of intention, readiness, and preparation to engage in a new behavior or action. This model has historically been applied to behavior modification and self-management, such as smoking cessation and weight loss. For example, a patient may engage in smoking behavior with little intention to stop. External influences, such as a primary care physician, may increase the patient's awareness of the harmful effects of this behavior, leading the patient to transition into a greater degree of readiness to stop. The patient may then engage in other activities to prepare to stop smoking, such as the use of medication or acupuncture. This model of health behavior has been used to understand and explain the natural history of decision-making for breast cancer reconstruction. Surgeons could consider using it as a decision-making framework for aesthetic surgery when contemplating a potential body-enhancement procedure. The model describes the surgical decision-making process along a continuum defined by four stages: pre-contemplation, contemplation, preparation, and action. **Fig. 1** describes the relationship between these stages of decision-making and the independent variables in the model.

With aesthetic surgery, the precontemplation stage is defined by either a lack of knowledge or lack of desire for cosmetic procedures. For example, a person with an aging face may have come across an article describing the use of Botox in alleviating the prominent frown lines associated with old age, setting the stage for research into this potential treatment avenue by this particular individual.

The contemplation stage is defined by thinking about and talking to others about cosmetic surgery. Patients in this stage are actively considering treatment issues and are motivated by higher levels of problem recognition, increasing knowledge, and changing attitudes. For example, patients in the contemplation stage may engage in role-playing that involves imagining their significant other's reaction to their body-contouring procedure. This can be a powerful motivator to proceeding to the next stage.

The preparation stage involves action-oriented activities motivated by the desire for an aesthetic change in appearance, such as obtaining a surgical consultation, evaluating treatment options, and learning about financial costs. This stage involves a greater readiness to undergo treatment and encompasses both cognitive and behavioral factors. The action stage is defined by receiving or not receiving surgery.

Health Belief Model

Several constructs from the Health Belief Model may affect the Stages of Change decision-making process for aesthetic surgery. Patient knowledge and attitudes play a central role across the continuum of decision-making. For example, among postpartum women, the transition to the contemplation stage could be motivated by increasing recognition that they have a problem with their rectus muscle diastasis and abdominal contour. Postpartum women may also become self-conscious over time about the physical appearance of their breasts, which may impact their sexuality. Or they may begin to feel inconvenienced by the clothing limitations from postpartum breast involution and/or ptosis. On the other hand, patient knowledge and attitudes may hinder consideration (contemplation) and initiation (preparation) of treatment. Limited knowledge about treatment effects, such as the restoration of body image and sexuality, may inhibit consideration. Concerns about the treatment outcomes, such as the impact of breast augmentation on mammography screening, may also deter consideration of cosmetic surgery.

External Influence Factors

External influence factors (physicians, significant others, family and/or friends, and media) play an important role in the knowledge and attitudes of patients, thereby influencing the decision-making process. The attitudes of primary care physicians and obstetricians and/or gynecologists, for example, can influence a woman in the contemplation stage for breast augmentation. For example, some

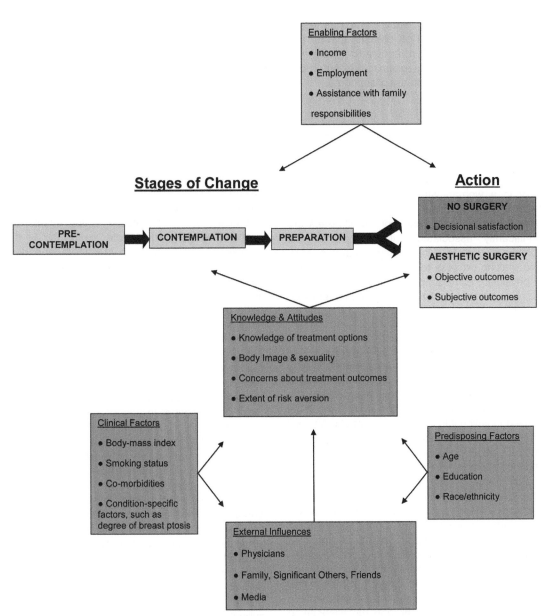

Fig. 1. The four stages of patient decision-making: precontemplation, contemplation, preparation, and action, and the effect of external variables on the patient.

physicians have misconceptions that breast implants are unsafe; these provider attitudes can impede a woman from moving from the contemplation to the preparation stage. In the preparation stage, the plastic surgeon–patient relationship can have a significant impact. For example, a woman who desires breast enhancement may have decided against it or delayed it because of a mismatch between the surgeon's and her own desired outcome or because of a lack of treatment choice between implant type, pocket location, incision location, or size. Family members can also play a crucial role, especially if they have experienced cosmetic surgery themselves. In addition, a significant other is a key component to this process. For example, a married woman may be less likely to be concerned about the scars from an augmentation-mastopexy compared with a woman who is not in a stable relationship. Finally, the media does have an influential role in transitioning women through the four stages. The negative press that breast implants received in the 1990s may slow a woman's progression to the preparation stage. On the other hand, the cultural pressure to reach ideal beauty standards (especially with the emphasis on breasts) that is reinforced by print, television, and radio media may facilitate a woman's progression to the contemplation stage for cosmetic breast procedures.

Clinical Factors

Clinical factors may also influence physician recommendations and patient attitudes toward surgery. For example, a physician may not be willing to perform an augmentation without mastopexy in a woman with grade 3 breast ptosis, despite her concerns about visible scarring. Obesity, nicotine use, and chronic illnesses are significantly associated with higher surgical complication rates, which may affect the decision-making process for the risk-adverse patient or physician. For example, a surgeon may not be willing to perform a rhytidectomy in a patient who uses nicotine.

Predisposing Factors

Predisposing factors influence a patient's knowledge and attitudes and, because the decision for aesthetic surgery is preference-sensitive, the decision will be heavily influenced by the cultural context in which it is made. For example, African-American and white individuals may have different attitudes toward sexuality, social relationships, and body image that lead to different decisions about cosmetic surgery. For example, African-Americans tend to place a greater emphasis on buttocks appearance, whereas whites are generally more concerned about breast aesthetics.[4] Other predisposing factors, such as age and education, may be associated with underlying attitudes and preferences that influence a patient's decisions about aesthetic surgery. For example, as women increase in age, receipt of cosmetic surgery increases. Age, through the association with knowledge, body image, and financial means, may play an important motivating role in the decision-making process.

Enabling Factors

Enabling factors are likely important issues influencing progression from contemplation to preparation and action. Socioeconomic status and access issues related to finances, availability of services, and the accommodation and acceptability of services may influence a patient's decision-making. In addition, having assistance with family responsibilities greatly enables the decision for elective surgery, especially among the postpartum population.

EVIDENCE-BASED CLINICAL ASSESSMENT: OBJECTIVE OUTCOMES
Major Complications

All would agree that major complications, such as hematomas, infections, and thromboembolic events, are unwanted adverse events, regardless of the type of surgery, and should be avoided. These types of complications can be life-threatening, lead to poor aesthetic outcomes, and result in financial burden for the patient. Outcomes related to major complications in aesthetic surgery are often limited to level 4 or 5 data from single-surgeon or single-center retrospective analyses. Because these are relatively rare events for aesthetic surgery, most data are limited in the sample size and power to identify independent risk factors associated with these complications. Large database analyses can overcome challenges in analyzing rare events and potentially underpowered studies through the availability of large patient samples treated by different providers in a variety of health care settings. However, most databases are related to insurance claims and, thus, are not applicable to aesthetic procedures. Two unique databases that contain information on aesthetic procedures are available to assess major complications in cosmetic surgery: Tracking Operations and Outcomes for Plastic Surgeons (TOPS) and CosmetAssure. TOPS was created by the American Society of Plastic Surgeons to monitor the quality of surgical care in plastic surgery. The advantage of TOPS is that it includes all types of operations, including cosmetic procedures. The disadvantage of TOPS is that it relies on voluntary self-reported data. CosmetAssure is an insurance policy sold nationally that covers medical and surgical complications associated with cosmetic surgery. As such, there is an incentive for participating surgeons to work with their patients who have a covered complication to submit claim information. However, the database does not include complications that are not covered by the insurance policy, such as infections that do not require intravenous antibiotics and wound dehiscence treated nonsurgically. These databases have been successfully used to assess postoperative complications among patients receiving breast augmentation and abdominoplasty.[5]

Condition-Specific Complications

Many complications with aesthetic surgery are condition-specific, such as capsular contracture with breast augmentation, intraabdominal injury with suction-assisted lipectomy, and facial nerve injury with rhytidectomy. Large databases are unlikely to collect condition-specific complications because they are not required to be reported by the American Society of Plastic Surgeons to TOPS and may not be a covered event under CosmetAssure. Another complicating factor is the time to the adverse event. Although facial nerve and intraabdominal injuries are acute events, complications such as capsular contracture or late breast seromas associated with anaplastic large cell lymphoma occur several years after surgery, and most studies have follow-up limited to 1 to 2 years postoperatively. Condition-specific complications may also be correlated to surgeon experience. However, the direction of this correlation is unclear. The relationship between high surgeon volume and low adverse event rates has been well-established in many areas of medicine.[6] One could also argue that highly experienced surgeons may be less risk adverse, use more aggressive techniques, and have better aesthetic outcomes but with more complications. Unfortunately, most outcomes research in cosmetic surgery represents the experience of a single surgeon and, as such, cannot be generalized to other surgeons with different levels of experience.

Revisional Surgery

Revisional surgery should be assessed when measuring aesthetic surgery outcomes because it represents an inadequate outcome with the original procedure. However, it is important to understand the potential shortcomings of measuring this outcome because it is inherently related to both patient and surgeon (1) satisfaction with the outcome and (2) willingness to proceed with further intervention. One could argue that revisional surgery is a good representation of dissatisfaction by both patient and physician. Rarely could one envision a revisional procedure if some level of dissatisfaction, although maybe to different degrees, was not present for both patient and surgeon. However, surgeons differ in their willingness to perform revisional surgery. Some surgeons believe that they did the best they could do for the patient at the time of the original surgery and are extremely reluctant to perform revisional surgery. Also, patients may seek revisional surgery from a different provider, which may not be captured when measuring outcomes from a single-surgeon experience.

Physical Functioning and Physical Dimensions

Objective measures of physical function are generally not measured for aesthetic procedures. Most outcomes with aesthetic surgery are related to quality of life, satisfaction, and subjective measures of physical functioning, although there are certain exceptions to this rule. Chest strength can be measured postoperatively with breast surgery, and visual field tests can be performed with upper lid blepharoplasty procedures.[7,8]

Objective measures of outcomes are not limited to physical functioning but can include changes in physical dimensions, especially with body-contouring procedures. Postoperative measurements of nipple position relative to sternal notch and inframammary folds confirm ptosis correction and breast symmetry with mastopexy. Preoperative and postoperative hip and waist dimensions confirm rectus abdominis muscle plication and excess tissue removal with abdominoplasty. Changes in extremity circumference dimensions demonstrate liposuction outcomes. Technologic advances in three-dimensional (3D) imaging should advance the objective assessment of changes in physical dimensions with aesthetic surgery. 3D technology can assess changes in breast projection, volume, shape, and position on the chest wall with breast augmentation, mastopexy, and reduction surgery.[9–11] Assessments can also be made with changes in the nasal dorsum, tip projection, and septal deviation with septorhinoplasty procedures.[12]

EVIDENCE-BASED CLINICAL ASSESSMENT: SUBJECTIVE OUTCOMES
Patient Satisfaction: Surgical Decision-Making Process

Medicine, and particularly aesthetic surgery, is a consumer-driven industry. As such, patient satisfaction is of primary importance. Two primary domains of patient satisfaction exist: (1) satisfaction with the surgical decision-making process and (2) satisfaction with the surgical outcome.

In regard to the decision for surgery, patients can have different levels of satisfaction with how that decision was made. Questions include: did the patient feel adequately informed of options, was the right decision made, would the same choices be made again, and did the patient have any regret? Two well-validated decision outcomes scales were proposed by Holmes-Rovner and O'Connor that are generic, not condition-specific, and are easily administered to any patient population.[13,14] These measures have been successfully used to measure outcomes in the post-mastectomy breast-reconstruction population[15] and are appropriate for the cosmetic patient. The BREAST-Q also has a validated measure of patient satisfaction with the surgical decision-making process for breast surgery that can be used in the reconstruction, reduction, mastopexy, and augmentation population.[16] In addition, the BREAST-Q has a validated measure of patient satisfaction with the amount of information the patient received preoperatively, the experience with the surgeon, and the experience with the nursing and office staff. Satisfaction outcomes can drive patient-centered process improvements and enhance the overall health care experience of the "consumer" patient. However, it is important to collect decisional satisfaction data near the time of the decision in order to avoid recall bias.

Satisfaction with the Surgical Outcome: Expert Opinion and the Patient Perspective

Traditionally, aesthetic outcomes have been assessed by physicians through the use of photographs. Key elements to this research approach are ensuring that (1) multiple experts assess the outcome, (2) the reviewers are blinded to the procedure, and (3) interrater reliability (ie, the degree of agreement among raters) is assessed.

Several statistical tools can be used to measure the concordance among raters, including Cohen's kappa, concordance correlation coefficient, and intraclass correlation. A high amount of disagreement among raters indicates either an inappropriate scale for measuring the outcome or lack of expertise by the raters. Unfortunately, there are many examples of poorly executed aesthetic outcomes studies in which bias was introduced into the study design by having only one expert, usually the treating physician, assess outcomes.

More recognition has recently been given to evaluating surgery outcomes from the perspective of the patient. This trend has coincided with patient-centric, consumer-driven health care. The validity of patient-reported outcome measures (PROMs) is dependent on the accuracy and reliability of the questions. When at all possible, previously validated, condition-specific measures, such as the Michigan Hand Questionnaire and BREAST-Q, should be used to assess outcomes from the patient's perspective. This ensures that the patient is accurately reporting on the concept of interest (ie, valid data) and that the results are reproducible (ie, reliable). Ad hoc questions can be used when validated PROMs are not available; however, these are at risk for being inaccurate and unreliable.[16,17] It is important to realize that, unlike satisfaction with the surgical decision-making process, satisfaction with surgical outcomes can change over time.[18] The appropriate time to assess satisfaction outcomes postoperatively is procedure-dependent. For example, one would expect satisfaction with breast augmentation to be the highest within the first 6 months postoperatively and gradually diminish overtime due to the occurrence of implant-related complications.

Health-Related Quality of Life

Changes in the quality of life of patients, along with patient satisfaction, are the primary measures of patient-reported outcomes. These outcomes capture the impact of a procedure on patients' daily activities in a clinically meaningful way using solid scientific techniques. Generic PROMs can be used to assess changes in patients' quality of life regardless of the type of procedure. However, condition-specific PROMs can often provide more meaningful clinical data. For example, the Medical Outcome Study Short Form 36-Item Health Survey is used to assess physical function through generic questions (eg, can a patient climb a set of stairs?).[19] However, the BREAST-Q, which is condition-specific to breast surgery, measures postoperative changes in patients' ability to move their arms and lift heavy objects.

Several health-related quality of life domains exist, including physical well-being, psychosocial well-being, and sexual well-being; and all are applicable to aesthetic surgery. For example, in regard to physical well-being, changes can be measured in nasal airways with rhinoplasty procedures,[20] in visual fields after blepharoplasty, and in activities of daily living that involve arm or trunk function after breast and abdominoplasty procedures. Furthermore, psychosocial and sexual well-being is intimately tied to aesthetic surgery. One can easily hypothesize the psychosocial impact of cosmetic facial surgery on professional promotions and workforce desirability for the aging population in competitive work environments. It is also easy to hypothesize a correlation between sexuality and cosmetic breast and body-contouring procedures for postpartum women.

When at all possible, a condition-specific PROM should be used to provide greater insight into the affect a procedure can have on quality of life. Unfortunately, validated PROMs are limited in aesthetic surgery. The BREAST-Q can be used to measure PROMs for aesthetic breast surgery; the Breast-Related Symptoms measure can be used to measure physical and psychosocial symptoms secondary to breast hypertrophy, and the Derriford Appearance Scale can be used to measure psychological distress and dysfunction secondary to aesthetic appearance problems.[21] Unfortunately, most PROMs for facial cosmetic surgery have limited scientific rigor in their development, validation, and content.[17]

LIMITATIONS WITH CURRENT EVIDENCE

Aesthetic surgery outcomes primarily have limitations with study design and measures. Almost all of the studies are retrospective case series producing level 4 or 5 data because the study designs do not attempt to control for the influence of confounding variables with consideration of the design of the study (eg, prospective) or the statistical analyses (eg, regression models). Most aesthetic surgery outcomes also represent the experience of a single surgeon and, as such, are limited in the ability to generalize results to other surgeons with different patient samples. In addition, many studies have limited follow-up and, therefore, do not assess outcomes long-term. Adequate follow-up is particularly important to evaluate the longevity of aesthetic procedures (eg, facial and breast surgery) and long-term complications related to devices (eg, breast implants).

Measures to assess aesthetic surgery outcomes are also limited. In general, current outcomes fall into one of two categories: the surgeon assesses the outcome or the surgeon asks the patient if they are satisfied; however, both measures are flawed. Objective assessment of outcomes by the provider should be performed by a blinded, expert panel to avoid observer bias. Patient-reported outcomes should be performed using validated, condition-specific measures. Unfortunately, condition-specific measures are limited for aesthetic procedures,[17] necessitating the use of generic measures that are able to provide general, not specific, information regarding patient satisfaction and quality of life. Use of ad hoc questions should be avoided when possible to ensure that the results are valid, reproducible, and comparable among different patient populations.[17]

FUTURE DIRECTIONS AND POLICY IMPLICATIONS

Many challenges exist with the assessment of aesthetic surgery outcomes. Perspectives on beauty vary by racial and/or ethnic background, geographic location, and socioeconomic status. Perspectives also vary between physician and patient. Thus, it is challenging to measure an outcome that varies by so many different factors. As a professional society, our goals for aesthetic surgery should include (1) ensuring patient safety, (2) advancing evidence-based aesthetic practices, and (3) regulating the delivery of aesthetic surgery through quality assessments.

Although there are substantial gaps in the scientific rigor of the data collecting process in aesthetic surgery, plastic surgeons have the opportunity to meet this need, improving patient safety and outcomes while distinguishing themselves as the national experts in this highly competitive market.

Future aesthetic surgery research goals need to address better measures and improved study designs. More condition-specific measures, such as the BREAST-Q, are needed to assess patient-reported outcomes from facial and body contouring procedures. Study designs need to be prospective, include multicenter or multisurgeon outcomes, incorporate blinded expert panels, and should address the issue of confounding variables through either study design or statistical analyses. Clinical registries are needed to assess long-term outcomes, which are particularly important for procedures to the breast involving implants and fat grafting. In addition, aesthetic surgery requires outcomes that include elements of value or cost in the analyses, such as comparative effectiveness and cost-effectiveness research. Decision analyses research can help surgeons manage difficult clinical problems that have significant financial risk for the patient with breast implants that need surveillance, are infected, or present with a seroma.

POLICY IMPLICATIONS

The assessment of aesthetic surgery outcomes still has the basic, yet fundamental, question to answer: whose perspective on outcomes—the patient or the physician—is of primary importance? Aesthetic surgery is an unusual physician-patient relationship in which the patient is the sole consumer of elective services with no third-party payer involvement. As a result, the traditional balance of power between the physician and patient has shifted toward the patient, which elevates the importance of patient's satisfaction with the surgical outcome. However, aesthetic surgery is highly unregulated. Surgeons and nonsurgeons from all types of educational backgrounds are engaging in aesthetic surgery. Anyone can claim to be a cosmetic surgeon, and the general public has little understanding of the necessary physician training required ensuring safe surgery and excellent outcomes. Therefore, expert opinion must be incorporated into the assessment of aesthetic surgery outcomes. Expert panels can establish outcome standards for aesthetic surgery that can provide public and consumer protection by confining practices to those individuals or groups who can meet acceptable standards.

SUMMARY

Plastic surgeons must be at the forefront of aesthetic surgery outcomes research. Evidence-based research is absolutely necessary to ensure high-quality care, and better study designs and measures will help create clinically meaningful outcomes.

REFERENCES

1. Chung KC, Swanson JA, Schmitz D, et al. Introducing evidence-based medicine to plastic and reconstructive surgery. Plast Reconstr Surg 2009; 123:1385–9.

2. Rohrich RJ, Eaves FF 3rd. So you want to be an evidence-based plastic surgeon? A lifelong journey. Plast Reconstr Surg 2011;127:467–72.

3. Montano D, Kasprzyk D, Taplin SH. The theory of reasoned action and the theory of planned behavior. In: Glanz K, Lewis FM, Rimer BK, editors. Health behavior and health education: theory, research, and practice. 2nd edition. San Francisco (CA): Jossey-Bass; 1997. p. 85–112.

4. Rubin L, Lemaine V, Pusic AL, et al. This reminds me of my struggle: breast reconstruction decisions among African-American women. Psychology and Health under review.

5. Alderman AK, Collins ED, Streu R, et al. Benchmarking outcomes in plastic surgery: national complication rates for abdominoplasty and breast augmentation. Plast Reconstr Surg 2009;124:2127–33.

6. Birkmeyer JD, Stukel TA, Siewers AE, et al. Surgeon volume and operative mortality in the United States [see comment]. N Engl J Med 2003;349:2117–27.

7. Cahill KV, Bradley EA, Meyer DR, et al. Functional indications for upper eyelid ptosis and blepharoplasty surgery: a report by the American Academy of Ophthalmology. Ophthalmology 2011;118:2510–7.

8. Battu VK, Meyer DR, Wobig JL. Improvement in subjective visual function and quality of life outcome measures after blepharoptosis surgery. Am J Ophthalmol 1996;121:677–86.

9. Eder M, v Waldenfels F, Sichtermann M, et al. Three-dimensional evaluation of breast contour and volume changes following subpectoral augmentation mammaplasty over 6 months. J Plast Reconstr Aesthet Surg 2011;64:1152–60.

10. Kovacs L, Eder M, Zimmermann A, et al. Three-dimensional evaluation of breast augmentation and the influence of anatomic and round implants on operative breast shape changes. Aesthetic Plast Surg 2012;36:879–87.

11. Henseler H, Smith J, Bowman A, et al. Objective evaluation of the latissimus dorsi flap for breast reconstruction using three-dimensional imaging. J Plast Reconstr Aesthet Surg 2012;65:1209–15.

12. Toriumi DM, Dixon TK. Assessment of rhinoplasty techniques by overlay of before-and-after 3D images. Facial Plast Surg Clin North Am 2011;19:711–23, ix.

13. Brehaut JC, O'Connor AM, Wood TJ, et al. Validation of a decision regret scale. Med Decis Making 2003;23:281–92.

14. Holmes-Rovner M, Kroll J, Schmitt N, et al. Patient satisfaction with health care decisions: the satisfaction with decision scale. Med Decis Making 1996;16:58–64.

15. Alderman AK, Hawley ST, Waljee J, et al. Understanding the impact of breast reconstruction on the surgical decision-making process for breast cancer. Cancer 2008;112:489–94.

16. Pusic AL, Klassen AF, Scott AM, et al. Development of a new patient-reported outcome measure for breast surgery: the BREAST-Q. Plast Reconstr Surg 2009;124:345–53.

17. Pusic AL, Lemaine V, Klassen AF, et al. Patient-reported outcome measures in plastic surgery: use and interpretation in evidence-based medicine. Plast Reconstr Surg 2011;127:1361–7.

18. Hu ES, Pusic AL, Waljee JF, et al. Patient-reported aesthetic satisfaction with breast reconstruction during the long-term survivorship Period. Plast Reconstr Surg 2009;124:1–8.

19. Ware JE Jr, Sherbourne CD. The MOS 36-item short-form health survey (SF-36). I. Conceptual framework and item selection. Med Care 1992;30:473–83.

20. Chaithanyaa N, Rai KK, Shivakumar HR, et al. Evaluation of the outcome of secondary rhinoplasty in cleft lip and palate patients. J Plast Reconstr Aesthet Surg 2011;64:27–33.

21. Collins ED, Kerrigan CL. Outcomes research: the path to evidence-based decisions in plastic surgery. In: Mathes SJ, editor. Plastic surgery. Philadelphia: Saunders; 2006. p. 35–50.

Measuring Outcomes in Craniofacial and Pediatric Plastic Surgery

Karen W.Y. Wong, MD, MSc, FRCSC[a],*,
Christopher R. Forrest, MD, MSc, FRCSC[a],
Tim E.E. Goodacre, MBBS, BSc, FRCS[b],
Anne F. Klassen, DPhil, BA[c]

KEYWORDS

- CLEFT-Q • Cleft lip and/or palate • Craniofacial surgery • Craniosynostosis
- Patient-reported outcomes • Health-related quality of life • Aesthetic outcomes

KEY POINTS

- The main goals of craniofacial and pediatric plastic surgery are to optimize function, aesthetic outcome, and health-related quality of life. These categories pose a considerable challenge in the measurement of outcomes from the patient perspective.
- Collection of comprehensive, clinically meaningful, and scientifically sound data is needed to determine best treatment plans as well as demonstrate quality of care for the purposes of advocacy and resource allocation.
- Patient-reported outcome (PRO) measurements reflect health concerns that patients describe as important. For patients with cleft lip and/or palate, the development of the CLEFT-Q has shown that there are several health concepts that have not been measured previously in the literature.
- PRO instruments should be developed with a global perspective for conditions that are prevalent worldwide. Cross-cultural adaptation may show that the same concept is expressed differently across cultures and a PRO instrument should reflect these differences.

INTRODUCTION

Craniofacial and pediatric plastic surgery encompass a wide variety of clinical presentations and conditions. Although the scope of practice of these two subspecialties is broad, there are concepts regarding the measurement of outcomes that pose similar challenges for craniofacial and general pediatric plastic surgeons. The management of clinical conditions such as cleft lip and/or palate (CLP) and craniosynostosis often begins in infancy and extends into adulthood. Treatment protocols vary widely and there may be procedures with competing goals within the same protocol. For example, it has been difficult to define a value for early palate repairs for optimal speech while taking into account the detrimental effects on facial growth. Determining the overall quality of care

Disclosures. None of the authors have any financial disclosures or conflicts of interest.
[a] Division of Plastic Surgery, Department of Surgery, Hospital for Sick Children, University of Toronto, 555 University Avenue, Toronto, ON M5G 1X8, Canada; [b] Clinical Medicine, The Spires Cleft Centre, Oxford Radcliffe Children's Hospital, University of Oxford, BAPRAS Professional Standards Committee, Headley Way, Headington, Oxford OX3 9DU, UK; [c] Department of Pediatrics, Clinical Epidemiology and Biostatistics, McMaster University, HSC 3N27, 1200 Main Street West, Hamilton, Ontario L8S 4J9, Canada
* Corresponding author. Division of Plastic and Reconstructive Surgery, Hospital for Sick Children, Suite 5431, 555 University Avenue, Toronto, ON M5G 1X8, Canada.
E-mail address: karenk.wong@utoronto.ca

Clin Plastic Surg 40 (2013) 305–312
http://dx.doi.org/10.1016/j.cps.2012.11.005
0094-1298/13/$ – see front matter © 2013 Elsevier Inc. All rights reserved.

delivered depends on the seemingly straightforward but challenging task of describing clinically meaningful outcomes.

Unlike many conditions in which the primary goal of treatment may be the resection of a tumor or treatment of an infection that may be evaluated more directly, the goals of treating congenital conditions such as CLP or craniosynostosis are to optimize function, aesthetic outcome, and health-related quality of life (HR-QL). The evaluation of outcomes is challenging because there is no established baseline to be restored for a patient with a congenital condition and surrogate outcomes, or measurements that are used as substitutes for a clinically meaningful endpoints,[1] are frequently used to describe final results. In addition, many of the conditions treated affect facial appearance. Having an appearance that "feels normal" has a significant influence on an individual's interpersonal interactions. Correcting bony and soft tissue facial features toward the norm is a cornerstone of craniofacial surgery; however, evaluating the success of this goal is also an important challenge. The patient perspective is a key component of defining outcomes in congenital conditions. Patient-reported outcomes (PROs) reflect the final endpoint of treatment, but have proven to be the most difficult to evaluate.

Careful consideration of the methods by which outcomes are measured is also increasingly important as the allocation of scarce resources becomes more dependent on the clinician's ability to prove that a treatment has had a beneficial effect. The management of many congenital conditions can be costly because of the large number of interventions required over a lengthy course of treatment, as in CLP, or because of the expense associated with innovative technology in surgical management, as in craniosynostosis.[2] From a broader perspective, the consideration of cost of care in concert with the associated outcomes is consistent across models of health care delivered around the world. Advocating for the best possible care for patients with congenital conditions in cost-focused environments requires clinicians to demonstrate measurable effects of treatment on patients from the functional, aesthetic, and HR-QL perspectives.

The aim of this article is to describe and justify the need for clinically meaningful and scientifically sound measurement of PROs. Challenges in the measurement of outcomes in craniofacial and pediatric plastic surgery are discussed first, with a focus on CLP and craniosynostosis. The role of meaningful measurements in the development of evidence-based guidelines and the definition of goals of treatment of these two conditions are then addressed, with a specific focus on CLP and the development of the CLEFT-Q, a new PRO instrument.

CHALLENGES IN MEASURING OUTCOMES IN CRANIOFACIAL AND PEDIATRIC PLASTIC SURGERY

There are unique challenges in measuring outcomes in craniofacial and pediatric plastic surgery patients. The most challenging aspects of surgical decision-making are frequently the difficulty presented by the options offered by different interactions between treatments and the complexity of measuring benefits associated with each. It is common to attribute such difficulties to the following:

1. The results of procedures performed in infancy do not become clear for several years and these results are not often reported in a standardized fashion
2. One of the primary goals of treatment is to improve aesthetic outcome and the measurement of this concept is challenging
3. A child represents a moving target with respect to measuring their patient perspective.

Ideally, a measurable outcome is a variable that can be assessed at the time of diagnosis or consultation to guide treatment decisions as well as evaluate surgical outcomes. Unfortunately, there are several domains of outcomes for which this is not possible in the pediatric congenital population. For example, a functional outcome such as speech is not measurable at the time of a primary cleft palate repair because the child has yet to learn to speak. The evaluation of such outcomes then necessarily occurs long after the initial procedure as a posttreatment audit tool alone and the measurement of change is not possible. Although this type of reporting of functional outcomes requires lengthy follow-up, outcomes such as speech, vision, or increased intracranial pressure are still more straightforward to evaluate than aesthetic or HR-QL outcomes; however, measuring a single functional outcome may not provide a complete reflection of the impact of the procedure. The reporting of functional outcomes in the literature is also highly variable due to the range of instruments used, making meta-analysis of study results difficult or impossible. Multicentered studies, such as Eurocleft and Americleft, have begun to introduce more standardized techniques of reporting to address this difficulty.[3,4] It is unlikely that a single outcome measure could ever be developed that would reflect accurately the results of a complete package of interventions. Therefore, coordinated efforts to adopt more comprehensive reporting techniques have been undertaken to address this challenge in complex conditions such as craniosynostosis.[5]

Defining Aesthetic Outcome in Infants and Children

One of the major aims of craniofacial surgery is to optimize the aesthetic appearance of the craniofacial region including a child's ability to show expression and spontaneous dynamic movement. In conditions such as facial palsy, for example, surgical decision-making includes many options such as complex reanimation of the paralyzed side of the face through an innervated microsurgically transferred muscle or weakening the contralateral side to create better symmetry. Defining just an aesthetic outcome for this condition requires at least a measure of symmetry and the patient's ability to express the desired emotion at rest and in motion; however, numerous other factors, including physical growth, will further complicate this evaluation. If the diverse causes of facial palsy (eg, congenital palsy, stroke, trauma, or tumor) are considered together with treatment side effects (eg, surgical scars or need for multiple procedures), some idea of the difficulty in evaluating outcomes robustly can be perceived.

Obtaining the Child's Perspective

Finally, obtaining the child or adolescent patient's perspective is perhaps one of the greatest methodological challenges in evaluating surgical outcomes. It is common to seek a proxy parent or caregiver report in place of the child's perspective when a child is too young, too ill, or cognitively impaired. However, a systematic review and several studies comparing the proxy and child assessments have shown that the correlation varies significantly.[6,7] In a study of children seeking pediatric, orthodontic, or craniofacial care, the rates of agreement between the child and the caregiver for oral HR-QL were found to be low-to-modest.[8] Children have shown to be able to self-report from age 6 years,[9] but a child's understanding of health concepts is less well understood.[10] A patient's perspective of their outcome will frequently change over time as their social environment changes, particularly during the early years. Children who begin school and, as a result, interact with several new individuals who may comment on their condition, may become more sensitive to their outcome than they were before school age. As they develop coping skills and social support networks, the

impact of their condition may change again. The concept of a changing "setpoint" has been a challenge in HR-QL research for some time and is termed *response shift*.[11] It is important to recognize this phenomenon and apply standard techniques and methodologies to first describe these changes and then to decipher their impact on the interpretation of final outcomes.[7,10] The development of PRO instruments for other conditions has shown that adaptations are necessary to accommodate the cognitive capabilities of the child over time.[12] As progress is made in developing scales for clinical use in different patient populations, addressing these methodological challenges will provide an understanding of how the child experiences their condition over time and explain how these changes should be accommodated in the measurement of outcomes.

DEFINING GOALS OF TREATMENT

As the scientific community engaged in improving cleft and craniofacial care continues to develop bodies of evidence to guide treatment decisions and improve quality of care, the measures adopted to assess PROs become even more important in the evaluation of the whole gamut of interventions delivered in a child's journey of care through to adulthood. Defining the goals of treatment in some conditions can be straightforward (eg, the restoration of occlusion following a fracture of the mandible); however, it is often more complex (eg, reshaping the cranial vault in craniosynostosis where improving HR-QL through functional and aesthetic changes is the goal). In complex cases, the completely objective isolated measurement of change of a functional or aesthetic variable may not reflect the overall goal of improving HR-QL. There is value to these individual measurements, but focusing on one or two specific outcomes may not provide a complete description of the affect of a surgical intervention on the patient.

The importance of defining clinically meaningful goals and then measuring these goals is highlighted using craniosynostosis as an example. For a single condition to be corrected, a family may be faced with options such as minimally invasive endoscopic approaches, open cranioplasty, distraction osteogenesis, and spring-assisted cranioplasty. The advantages and disadvantages of each technique may manifest in different types of outcomes. Most studies reported to date are case series or retrospective case reviews and there is great value in these reports from experts despite the apparent low level of evidence.[13] The challenge lies in comparing these reports to each other, especially when the benefits of one procedure compared with another may be found in a different outcome, such as decreased operative time or decreased burden of care. In addition, surgical success has often been defined in terms of lower complication or reoperation rates and, although these variables are important surrogate outcomes, the impact of surgery on patients is not well represented.[14,15] For example, the Whitaker scale provides an indication of the need for further surgery and the extent of subsequent treatment, and it is valuable for these reasons. However, this scale represents a surrogate, subjective measurement made from variable perspectives (the patient, the surgeon, and the family) that may not consistently show the impact of a cranioplasty on the patients themselves.[16] Szpalski and colleagues[5] have outlined a comprehensive set of outcomes commonly used in the management of craniosynostosis that includes a range of functional and aesthetic concerns. The complexity of the condition and its treatment is reflected in the wide variety of outcome categories, which include radiographic studies, otolaryngology, ophthalmology, dentistry and orthodontics, neurologic development, and quality of life assessments. The aesthetic outcome from procedures is often analyzed using craniometric measurements and, although these variables provide important insight into surgical techniques, these measures may not reflect the actual aesthetic impact of the procedure. These investigators also identify the need for the development of comprehensive PRO instruments to complement the array of specific physically determined metrics, to put these outcomes into a practical and useful context for treatment decision-making.

As the surgical techniques used in the management of craniosynostosis evolve, measuring a comprehensive set of outcomes that include the patient perspective should help to provide a more value-based assessment of the advantages and disadvantages of each technique. For example, a recent study showed that children undergoing a longer surgery with increased exposure to inhaled anesthetics had lower neurodevelopmental scores.[17] This finding could have implications on the type of surgery selected for a patient if the association is proven to be causal. However, there may be other variables that explain this outcome, such as the severity of the initial cranial deformity and the impact of that deformity on the brain preoperatively. If the benefit of the aesthetic outcome of these procedures is not found to outweigh the risk of neurodevelopmental delay, surgical decision-making might follow a different path. Establishing the balance between different outcomes is complex. First, proving that the association is causal in this case would require a randomized controlled trial, controlling for other confounding variables that would be identified in a comprehensive assessment of outcomes. Second, comparing the benefit of the aesthetic outcome to the risk of neurodevelopmental delay would require well-defined outcome measures of aesthetic results beyond craniometric measurements alone.

AN EXAMPLE CONDITION: CLEFT LIP AND PALATE

As discussed above, evaluating functional and aesthetic outcomes using objective measures alone does not provide an assessment of the impact of treatment on patients. The Eurocleft study highlighted the importance of including the patient perspective by showing that patient and parent satisfaction with cleft care, measured using an ad hoc questionnaire, did not correlate with objective outcome measures.[18] This may be attributed to the methodology of the ad hoc questionnaire, which was not designed to accurately measure concepts in this population. More plausibly, there is some validity in the findings and, therefore, concern that patients and their families do not consistently experience a positive impact from the invasive procedures performed. Cleft care is complex and involves a multidisciplinary team of care providers, similar to craniosynostosis management as described above. The comprehensive approach to describing outcomes outlined by Szpalski and colleagues[5] that includes the patient perspective provides a useful framework that can be adapted for CLP.

Functional Outcomes in CLP

Functional outcomes in CLP include appearance, speech, dentition, feeding, hearing, and breathing. Whereas there are advanced methods of evaluating these functions within each of these specialties, the variety of outcome instruments reported in the literature limit the potential for comparison between studies. There have been some advances in standardization of measures, an example being the measurement of dental arch development. The Eurocleft and Americleft studies both used the GOSLON Yardstick to evaluate growth disturbance of the dental arch and maxilla,[19,20] alongside the detailed cephalometric measurements that have long been used in the assessment of maxillary hypoplasia and occlusal deformities.[21,22] The assessment of speech, in which the perceptual assessment of an expert speech-language pathologist remains the gold standard to detect abnormalities, is more difficult to standardize. The GOSSPAS standard has been widely adopted across Europe for interunit comparison, but, as a consequence, the variety of other measures used around the world has weakened the evidence base for predictive value. There have been efforts to coordinate the reporting of speech outcomes in patients with CLP across languages.[23] More specifically, a recent systematic review of the efficacy of speech interventions in this population found that the inconsistency in the reporting of outcomes, in addition to the variety of interventions and the risk of bias, limited the ability to draw conclusions despite the fact that 6 of the 17 studies evaluated were randomized controlled trials.[24] The measurement of functional outcomes within each specialty involved in cleft care is becoming more consistent as the reporting of clinical standards in countries becomes mandated from a policy perspective, such as in the United Kingdom.

Aesthetic Outcomes in CLP

Aesthetic outcomes present another major challenge in the evaluation of the treatment of CLP. In a recent systematic review of aesthetic outcome measures for patients with CLP, Sharma and colleagues[25] outline several different strategies used for the assessment of aesthetic outcome, namely clinical, photographic, video, and three-dimensional evaluations. Although the techniques of assessment differ, the type of measurement used in each of these strategies is similar, with most using a five-point scale. It is common to report results of these assessments in a descriptive manner. However, the implication of the findings of these assessments to clinical practice, or assigning clinical meaning to the evaluations, has been more difficult to discern. Although several outcome measures have been subjected to traditional psychometric tests of validity and reliability, these tests generate scales that typically provide ordinal, rather than interval-level, data (subsequent levels in a given scale may not be equally spaced apart in "difficulty," so standard statistical analyses should not be applied). As a result, the findings are less likely to reflect clinical change accurately.

Modern psychometric methods, such as Rasch analysis, approach the assessment of PROs by assigning a probability to a certain pattern of an individual patient's answers on a scale developed using methods that create through interval-level measurement. Thus, the measurement of aesthetic outcomes may become more clinically significant and applicable to that patient when modern psychometric methods are used.[26] Creating meaningful measurement in aesthetic outcomes in

patients with CLP also depends on the specific goal. If the goal is to remove the stigma of CLP (ie, achieve "normal"), defining an aesthetic threshold of acceptability, as opposed to a rating scale, would be beneficial. However, if the goal is to improve appearance, a rating scale with well-defined interval-level measurement would be useful. It is also likely that a combination of perspectives need to be sought (eg, experienced clinician, patient, and general public) to understand the aesthetic outcome as well as guide treatment decisions. However, it should also be undeniable that the principle goal of treatment is to improve the patient's own perception of their appearance and well-being, and this perspective should guide the judgment of all treatment options.

Outcomes of All Facets of CLP

Evaluating all facets of outcomes beyond aesthetics would benefit from clinically meaningful measurement from the patient's perspective. Although it is more obvious that the patient perspective is the most important in the assessment of the psychosocial impact of their condition and its treatment, it is arguable that the most important perspective in the evaluation of both functional and aesthetic outcomes is also that of the patient.[27] Collecting PRO data is an essential component of outcome evaluation because these data represent the most clinically relevant results. To ensure that this approach is done in a manner that addresses the concerns and challenges raised above, the methodology behind PRO instrument development and validation needs to be robust and to follow established guidelines.[28]

CLEFT-Q: DEVELOPMENT OF A PRO INSTRUMENT

In a systematic review of PRO instruments used in pediatric plastic surgery, six different generic instruments were found to have been used, with five of them having been determined to be scientifically sound.[29] Generic instruments are designed to enable comparisons of populations of patients, and the clinical meaning or concepts important to any single population may not be captured in the measurements. Eight different condition-specific instruments assessing quality of life in pediatric plastic surgery populations were identified, with six of these using the patient report instead of a proxy. Only one of these instruments, the YQOL-FD, was developed according to international guidelines for instrument development and could be highly recommended for use. Importantly, the YQOL was also the only instrument developed with patient input, with the remainder being developed using expert opinion, existing measures, and a review of the literature.

Patients with CLP experience their condition and the impact of its treatment in a unique fashion. Patient input is an integral component of item generation in instrument development because it identifies health concerns that patients believe to be important. The YQOL, which has modules for facial differences and craniofacial surgery, is a PRO measure for the assessment of quality of life. It addresses the domains of negative consequences, negative self-image, stigma, positive consequences, and coping.[30] Although it is well designed to measure these domains, it does not assess the patient's perspective of their functional outcomes.

In seeking to evaluate PROs in patients with CLP, the authors were unable to find an instrument developed using the gold standard methods of PRO instrument development for this population. The authors are developing such an instrument for patients with CLP, called the CLEFT-Q, using previously published methodology.[28] In the first phase, a conceptual framework for the health concepts that should be measured in the population are identified through a systematic review of the literature,[31] in-depth qualitative patient interviews, and expert opinion. An exhaustive list of potential items assessing each concept within the framework is then created, using the patients' own words whenever possible. In the second phase of item reduction, a preliminary version of the instrument is field-tested on a large population of patients to determine which questions are the most effective in measuring the health concepts. The third and final phase includes further psychometric evaluation to examine the measurement properties of the final instrument.

Conceptual Framework for Patient Interviews

In a systematic review of the literature, the authors did not identify any patient-reported outcome measures designed specifically for CLP.[31] The patient perspective has been measured previously in 26 studies of patients with CLP using 29 different instruments, including three generic instruments designed for use in the general population. Because the health concerns of this population are unique, measuring change with treatment is unlikely to be captured using instruments that were designed for use in other patient populations. Patients with CLP were included in the group of adolescents interviewed in the development of the YQOL, but this group also included patients with acquired facial differences from burns or

trauma.[30] Based on the concepts that had been measured previously in the literature, the authors developed a preliminary conceptual framework to guide subsequent patient interviews. The main domains of the preliminary framework included physical, psychological, and social health.

The authors then performed 53 interviews with patients in three high-income, English-speaking countries (Canada, United States, and United Kingdom). These individual in-depth interviews were analyzed using the qualitative methodology of interpretive description.[32] Line-by-line coding was performed to develop health concepts important in this patient population. From this analysis, the authors identified several concepts that arose that had not previously been measured. The expanded conceptual framework included the following domains:

- Appearance
- Physical health
- Social health
- Psychological health
- Treatment and recovery
- Process of care.

Within these domains, the concepts were expressed in a manner specific to patients with CLP. Rather than simply expressing satisfaction with the nose, for example, patients used phrases such as "my nose is flat" or "one side of my nose is bigger than the other." Patients expressed overall satisfaction with their appearance in terms of different scenarios, using phrases such as "I only take pictures from one side" or "I don't like the way I look in pictures." These comments provide some insight into why direct questions such as "how satisfied are you with your overall appearance" may not capture the nuances of a patient's perspective, change over time, or change with treatments.

Age Range of Patients

The CLEFT-Q is being developed as a self-report PRO instrument for young patients from age 6 to 22 years. This range was chosen to first describe any findings of response shift over time or with treatments, and then to take these changes into consideration in the development of scales. Based on these findings, it is unlikely that a single scale will apply to patients across all ages and that we will need several modules targeted at different age groups. Rigorous psychometric analysis in the developmental stage of the CLEFT-Q will maximize its clinical applicability in the future across a patient's journey from childhood to adolescence.

Economic Status and Cultural Variation Among Patients

CLP and other congenital conditions are often more prevalent in low-income and middle-income countries in comparison with high-income countries.[33] The burden of CLP is arguably greater in these countries where access to care is limited. Advocating for this patient population worldwide depends on our ability to better define this burden. An instrument such as the CLEFT-Q would be useful in showing the impact of having CLP, as well as treatment, in patients from these countries. As the scientific community moves forward with defining outcomes from a comprehensive perspective, it is important to consider the global patient population. Cross-cultural adaptation of PRO measures is a complex process that requires the consideration of linguistic and cultural variation. The linguistic translation of a measure developed in a high-income country for use in a low-income country may not provide accurate and clinically meaningful measurement. Using the example in the discussion describing patients' expression of their overall satisfaction with appearance, it may be that patients in lower income countries do not frequently have their photos taken and they may use other phrases to describe their appearance. Patients in high-income countries may report the impact of a fistula as an inability to play a wind instrument in music classes, whereas patients in low-income and middle-income countries may not have this opportunity in school or may even not be attending school. In developing the CLEFT-Q such that the measure will be applicable to a global population, the team has performed in-depth qualitative interviews in three low-income countries (ie, India, Kenya, and the Philippines) in collaboration with local surgeons and international organizations. Preliminary analysis of these data further supports the need to seek the patient perspective broadly because the manifestation of certain outcomes varies based on culture in addition to language.

SUMMARY

Craniofacial and pediatric plastic surgery present important challenges in the measurement of outcomes. Evaluating the goals of optimizing function, aesthetic outcome, and HR-QL in a pediatric population requires complex methodology in the evolving science of measurement. Comprehensive outcome evaluation is a necessary step in showing the value of surgical interventions and it is essential that, in the future, this includes reports from the patients' perspectives. To portray accurately this value, the development of PRO instruments should follow scientifically sound and clinically meaningful measurement techniques. The initial stages of development of the CLEFT-Q show that there are health concepts that patients describe as being important that have not been measured in the past, and that these concepts are expressed differently based on language and culture. As the current environment of cost-focused, value-based resource allocation for health care develops, employing a comprehensive array of outcomes will be useful in advocating for the craniofacial and pediatric plastic surgery patient population.

REFERENCES

1. D'Agostino RB Jr. Debate: the slippery slope of surrogate outcomes. Curr Control Trials Cardiovasc Med 2000;1(2):76–8.
2. Thoma A, Ignacy TA. Health services research: impact of quality of life instruments on craniofacial surgery. J Craniofac Surg 2012;23(1):283–7.
3. Semb G, Brattstrom V, Molsted K, et al. The Eurocleft study: intercenter study of treatment outcome in patients with complete cleft lip and palate. Part 1: introduction and treatment experience. Cleft Palate Craniofac J 2005;42(1):64–8.
4. Long RE Jr, Hathaway R, Daskalogiannakis J, et al. The Americleft study: an inter-center study of treatment outcomes for patients with unilateral cleft lip and palate part 1. Principles and study design. Cleft Palate Craniofac J 2011;48(3):239–43.
5. Szpalski C, Weichman K, Sagebin F, et al. Need for standard outcome reporting systems in craniosynostosis. Neurosurg Focus 2011;31(2):E1.
6. Eiser C, Morse R. Can parents rate their child's health-related quality of life? Results of a systematic review. Qual Life Res 2001;10(4):347–57.
7. De Civita M, Regier D, Alamgir AH, et al. Evaluating health-related quality-of-life studies in paediatric populations: some conceptual, methodological and developmental considerations and recent applications. Pharmacoeconomics 2005;23(7):659–85.
8. Wilson-Genderson M, Broder HL, Phillips C. Concordance between caregiver and child reports of children's oral health-related quality of life. Community Dent Oral Epidemiol 2007;35(Suppl 1):32–40.
9. Riley AW. Evidence that school-age children can self-report on their health. Ambul Pediatr 2004;4(Suppl 4):371–6.
10. Bevans KB, Riley AW, Moon J, et al. Conceptual and methodological advances in child-reported outcomes measurement. Expert Rev Pharmacoecon Outcomes Res 2010;10(4):385–96.
11. Sprangers MA, Schwartz CE. Integrating response shift into health-related quality of life research: a theoretical model. Soc Sci Med 1999;48(11):1507–15.

12. Ravens-Sieberer U, Erhart M, Wille N, et al. Generic health-related quality-of-life assessment in children and adolescents: methodological considerations. Pharmacoeconomics 2006;24(12):1199–220.

13. Sackett DL, Rosenberg WM, Gray JA, et al. Evidence based medicine: what it is and what it isn't. BMJ 1996;312(7023):71–2.

14. Seruya M, Oh AK, Boyajian MJ, et al. Long-term outcomes of primary craniofacial reconstruction for craniosynostosis: a 12-year experience. Plast Reconstr Surg 2011;127(6):2397–406.

15. Lee HQ, Hutson JM, Wray AC, et al. Analysis of morbidity and mortality in surgical management of craniosynostosis. J Craniofac Surg 2012;23(5):1256–61.

16. Whitaker LA, Bartlett SP, Schut L, et al. Craniosynostosis: an analysis of the timing, treatment, and complications in 164 consecutive patients. Plast Reconstr Surg 1987;80(2):195–212. http://dx.doi.org/10.1111/j.1460-9592.2012.03843.x. [Epub ahead of print].

17. Naumann HL, Haberkern CM, Pietila KE, et al. Duration of exposure to cranial vault surgery: associations with neurodevelopment among children with single-suture craniosynostosis. Paediatr Anaesth 2012.

18. Semb G, Brattstrom V, Molsted K, et al. The Eurocleft study: intercenter study of treatment outcome in patients with complete cleft lip and palate. Part 4: relationship among treatment outcome, patient/parent satisfaction, and the burden of care. Cleft Palate Craniofac J 2005;42(1):83–92.

19. Molsted K, Brattstrom V, Prahl-Andersen B, et al. The Eurocleft study: intercenter study of treatment outcome in patients with complete cleft lip and palate. Part 3: dental arch relationships. Cleft Palate Craniofac J 2005;42(1):78–82.

20. Hathaway R, Daskalogiannakis J, Mercado A, et al. The Americleft study: an inter-center study of treatment outcomes for patients with unilateral cleft lip and palate part 2. Dental arch relationships. Cleft Palate Craniofac J 2011;48(3):244–51.

21. Brattstrom V, Molsted K, Prahl-Andersen B, et al. The Eurocleft study: intercenter study of treatment outcome in patients with complete cleft lip and palate. Part 2: craniofacial form and nasolabial appearance. Cleft Palate Craniofac J 2005;42(1):69–77.

22. Daskalogiannakis J, Mercado A, Russell K, et al. The Americleft study: an inter-center study of treatment outcomes for patients with unilateral cleft lip and palate part 3. Analysis of craniofacial form. Cleft Palate Craniofac J 2011;48(3):252–8.

23. Henningsson G, Kuehn DP, Sell D, et al. Universal parameters for reporting speech outcomes in individuals with cleft palate. Cleft Palate Craniofac J 2008;45(1):1–17.

24. Bessell A, Sell D, Whiting P, et al. Speech and language therapy interventions for children with cleft palate: a systematic review. Cleft Palate Craniofac J 2012. http://dx.doi.org/10.1597/11-20. [Epub ahead of print].

25. Sharma VP, Bella H, Cadier MM, et al. Outcomes in facial aesthetics in cleft lip and palate surgery: a systematic review. J Plast Reconstr Aesthet Surg 2012;65(9):1233–45.

26. Pusic AL, Lemaine V, Klassen AF, et al. Patient-reported outcome measures in plastic surgery: use and interpretation in evidence-based medicine. Plast Reconstr Surg 2011;127(3):1361–7.

27. Porter ME. What is value in health care? N Engl J Med 2010;363(26):2477–81.

28. Cano SJ, Klassen A, Pusic AL. The science behind quality-of-life measurement: a primer for plastic surgeons. Plast Reconstr Surg 2009;123(3):98e–106e.

29. Klassen AF, Stotland MA, Skarsgard ED, et al. Clinical research in pediatric plastic surgery and systematic review of quality-of-life questionnaires. Clin Plast Surg 2008;35(2):251–67.

30. Patrick DL, Topolski TD, Edwards TC, et al. Measuring the quality of life of youth with facial differences. Cleft Palate Craniofac J 2007;44(5):538–47.

31. Klassen AF, Tsangaris E, Forrest CR, et al. Quality of life of children treated for cleft lip and/or palate: a systematic review. J Plast Reconstr Aesthet Surg 2012;65(5):547–57.

32. Thorne S, Kirkham SR, MacDonald-Emes J. Interpretive description: a noncategorical qualitative alternative for developing nursing knowledge. Res Nurs Health 1997;20(2):169–77.

33. Mossey PA, Little J, Munger RG, et al. Cleft lip and palate. Lancet 2009;374(9703):1773–85.

Measuring Outcomes in Hand Surgery

Aviram M. Giladi, MD[a], Kevin C. Chung, MD, MS[b],*

KEYWORDS

- Patient-reported outcomes • Hand surgery outcomes • Patient-reported measures of hand function
- COSMIN • CAT • PROMIS • Health services research

KEY POINTS

- A shift towards value-based insurance models has begun with programs designed to reduce patient costs and increase access and use of high-value treatments, while discouraging low-value treatments.
- It is important to choose the questionnaire(s) that will suit the study needs.
- In addition, the investigator must be careful to avoid overburdening subjects with numerous tests and questionnaires.
- Finding the right combination of outcomes metrics without compromising study quality can be facilitated in part by thoughtful selection of robust and appropriate instruments.
- As the use of item response theory and computerized adaptive testing continues to mold the future of health services and outcomes research, measuring outcomes in hand surgery will again require a shift in technique, metric design, and study execution.

OVERVIEW

The upper extremity is a highly specialized functional, sensory, and aesthetic unit. The upper extremity can also suffer a unique range of insults. In 2010, the United States Bureau of Labor Statistics reported the annual incidence of hand injuries at 25.1 per 10,000 workers, and the most frequently injured population were young, active workers.[1] When the costs of medical care, rehabilitation, and productivity loss are computed for this younger population of patients with trauma as well as the often older population with arthritis, neuropathies, and other sources of pain and functional loss, the burden of hand disorders is massive.[2] How providers evaluate and manage hand disorders is critical to individuals and to society.

On the national level, as health care delivery and reimbursement in the United States undergoes rapid and substantial change, the focus on quality and value of care continues to increase. A shift towards value-based insurance models has begun.[3,4] These programs aim to reduce patient costs and increase access and use of high-value

Disclosures: None.
Supported in part by grants from the National Institute on Aging and National Institute of Arthritis and Musculoskeletal and Skin Diseases (R01 AR062066) and from the National Institute of Arthritis and Musculoskeletal and Skin Diseases (2R01 AR047328-06) and a Midcareer Investigator Award in Patient-Oriented Research (K24 AR053120) (to Dr Kevin C. Chung).
[a] Section of Plastic Surgery, Department of Surgery, The University of Michigan Health System, 1500 East Medical Center Drive, Ann Arbor, MI 48109-5340, USA; [b] Section of Plastic Surgery, The University of Michigan Medical School, 2130 Taubman Center, SPC 5340, 1500 East Medical Center Drive, Ann Arbor, MI 48109-5340, USA
* Corresponding author. Section of Plastic Surgery, University of Michigan Health System, 2130 Taubman Center, SPC 5340, 1500 East Medical Center Drive, Ann Arbor, MI 48109-5340.
E-mail address: kecchung@umich.edu

treatments, while discouraging low-value treatments. Choosing Wisely and other similar campaigns are also emphasizing appropriate and evidence-based surgical interventions.[5] Fee-for-service reimbursement is changing, and quality of care will play an increasing role in provider compensation.[6,7] These developments have resulted in a renewed focus on the need for high-quality evidence to support provider decision making and delivery of care.

In the United States, Canada, the United Kingdom, and many other nations, health services research has been a substantial area of focus for more than 15 years.[8,9] This field analyzes how patients access health care, what care costs, and what outcomes the patients experience as a result of this care. As work in this area continues to increase, the volume of literature addressing challenging issues in treatment quality, value, effectiveness, and appropriateness is growing. However, the quality of this literature is inconsistent. Interpreting the various results and their potential impact also continues to be a challenge. Considering the volume of hand disorders in the United States and worldwide, providing high-quality, sustainable, effective, and cost-conscious care is paramount. Especially when preparing for the changing landscape of health care, an awareness of the various factors affecting outcomes after hand surgery is critical for continued improvement and success.

PATIENT-REPORTED OUTCOMES IN HAND SURGERY

When evaluating the quality of care in hand surgery, standard functional metrics have traditionally been measured: fracture healing, range of motion, strength, sensation, and others.[10-12] However, in many cases, what providers consider substantial improvement does not align with the perceptions and experiences of patients.[13,14] That is not to say that traditional objective metrics cannot show significant differences in outcomes; rather, what is measured by these functional tests often does not translate to the outcomes desired by the patient, provider, or society. For example, fracture union on radiograph does not always equate with a patient having high satisfaction with their outcome or with returning to activities of daily living (ADL). A growing appreciation of this dichotomy has led the drive to using patient-reported outcome (PRO) metrics in the assessment of upper extremity disease. PRO questionnaires allow providers to assess function, health-related quality-of-life (HRQL), and satisfaction from the patient's perspective.[15,16]

Understanding of a patient's HRQL requires an appreciation of physical, mental, and social well-being.[17] How satisfaction, function, pain control, and other components can affect HRQL has a substantial impact on treatment decisions and outcomes. In addition, the degree to which expenditures can be justified is guided by the expected improvement in HRQL. Improving the way these components are measured has formed the basis for design, application, and evaluation of numerous PRO instruments. The design and refinement of a PRO instrument is a difficult task, requiring a mix of qualitative and quantitative assessments. It must be tested with pilot patient cohorts, and complex statistical analysis is needed to determine reliability and consistency. The instrument must then be evaluated for validity and responsiveness for the disease-state in question, which requires that each new metric be examined for each specific subset of patients the investigators intend to evaluate. The details of this process, and the various statistical measurements that are used, have been described by numerous investigators and are not covered in detail here.[15,18-21] **Table 1** contains a list of key quality domains and definitions.

CHOOSING AN OUTCOMES INSTRUMENT

Even when properly vetted, validated PRO metrics do not all perform at the same level. For example, the Michigan Hand Questionnaire (MHQ)[22] and the Disability of Arm, Shoulder, and Hand (DASH) questionnaire[23] have both been validated for patients with carpal tunnel syndrome (CTS)[24]; however, with additional subdomains geared towards more than just functional aspects of disease, the MHQ is better able to evaluate the symptomatic components of CTS.[24] Another example is the Short Form-36 (SF-36)[25] that has been validated for rheumatoid arthritis (RA).[26,27] For patients with RA, DASH scores were highly correlated with SF-36 for pain, but DASH was only moderately correlated for physical and mental function.[28] In contrast, for patients after distal radius fracture fixation, MHQ and DASH are significantly more responsive than SF-36.[29,30] The challenge in hand surgery is deciding which metrics should be used for each patient population. Although the number of available PROs continues to grow, the number of valid and robust outcomes measures remains few and inconsistently used.[10,31] Appropriate selection of PRO metrics governs the value of any study results.

PRO INSTRUMENTS

PRO questionnaires are classified as general, system specific, and disease specific.[21] General

Table 1
Definitions for key measurement properties used in evaluating the quality of patient-reported outcomes instruments

Measurement Property	Definition
Content validity	The degree to which the content of an instrument is an adequate reflection of the construct to be measured
Criterion validity	Strength of relationship between questionnaire scores and a measurable external criterion (the gold standard)
Construct validity	The degree to which the scores of a questionnaire are consistent with the theoretic construct (hypothesis) that is being measured
Face validity	The degree to which items in an instrument look as though they are an adequate reflection of the construct being measured
Internal consistency	The extent to which the items are interrelated, and thus measure the same construct
Reliability	The extent to which patients can be distinguished from each other despite measurement errors
Test-retest reliability	The extent to which scores for patients who have not changed are the same in repeated measurements over time
Inter-rater reliability	The extent to which scores for patients who have not changed are the same over repeated measurements by different examiners during the same visit
Responsiveness	The ability to detect clinically meaningful change over time in the construct being measured
Interpretability	The degree to which quantitative scores can be given qualitative meaning. Identifying clinically important differences in results
Cross-cultural equivalence	The same measurement instrument used in different cultures measures the same construct without additional external cultural influences on results

PRO measures evaluate qualitative and quantitative aspects of the patient's life without focusing on any specific disease or organ system. They ascertain general well-being, including components of pain, vitality, emotional and mental health, and self-assessment of ability to perform daily functions and activities. The SF-36 and Arthritis Impact Measurement Scales 2 (AIMS2)[32] are frequently used general PRO measures in hand surgery outcomes research.

System-specific, or domain-specific, instruments focus on an organ system or functional unit. These PRO metrics are geared toward better understanding of how the specific system of interest is affected by a disease state, what effects this has on the patient, and how these problems improve after intervention, which makes domain-specific instruments more valuable in intervention trials, but less likely to detect broader features of health states.[15] The most commonly used instruments in upper extremity studies are the MHQ, DASH, and Patient-rated Wrist Evaluation (PRWE) outcomes questionnaire.[19,33]

Disease-specific instruments are geared toward a population grouped by a particular disorder. These metrics are used in evaluating treatment of the specific disease. The focused nature of the questionnaire often results in high responsiveness when used in the appropriate patient population.[15] However, the design often limits use in evaluating other diseases, even within the same system, which restricts how the results from a disease-specific instrument are used. The Carpal Tunnel Questionnaire (CTQ) is a commonly used disease-specific instrument.[34]

For PRO metrics of all types, it is important to consider cross-cultural applications as well. Validity and responsiveness are population dependent, and this is an even greater issue when the different populations of interest do not speak the same language or live with similar cultural norms. The process of translating and subsequently validating quantitative and PRO instruments is challenging. It not only requires language conversion but also ensuring that subtle nuances and organizational aspects of the translated questionnaire do not adversely affect the way patients understand and answer questions.[35–37] This can be something as clear as Korean patients showing limited understanding of questions related to self-feeding with a spoon rather than using chopsticks.[38] It can also be more complex, such as loss of idiomatic quality in translation from English to Spanish resulting in patients perceiving the questionnaire as less serious.[39] The details of these concepts are beyond the scope of this article. However, as health care delivery and research becomes increasingly global, instruments with adequate cross-cultural equivalence will have broader usability in patient care and health services research.

UNDERSTANDING THE LITERATURE ON PRO METRIC QUALITY

Understanding the classification scheme discussed earlier is only a small part of the decision tree in selecting outcomes tools. Adequate consistency, reliability, validity, and responsiveness of the instrument are a large component of this decision process as well. Although the volume of literature evaluating these quality measures of the different PRO metrics continues to increase, understanding these studies and the quality of their results remains challenging for most. Making this even more problematic, definitions and usage of terms are inconsistent across various studies, which results in difficult decision making

in planning a PRO-focused study, and limits the quality of methodology and content of systematic reviews.[40]

A common concern when using PRO measures is how to interpret the scores. For example, what does a 10-point difference in the MHQ after treatment really mean; it is statistically significant, but is it clinically significant? Interpretability provides an indication as to how well the quantitative data can be translated into qualitatively (clinically) relevant results.[41] This is most often done by determining the minimal clinically important difference (MCID).[42] In patients with CTS, the MCID of the MHQ pain subdomain is 23, whereas the MCID for the function subdomain is 13.[43] For patients with RA, the MHQ subdomain MCID for pain is 11 and for function it is 13.[43] Although useful when available, the applicability is limited because meaningful clinical change varies between patient groups. However, having the MCID for a questionnaire in the population being evaluated gives an indication as to the clinical relevance of study results.

An additional approach to addressing the challenges in PRO metric evaluation has been to set guidelines and quality standards. Terwee and colleagues[44] published quality criteria for measurement properties (**Table 2**), and provided

Table 2
Quality criteria for the key measurement properties used in evaluating patient-reported outcomes instruments

Measurement Property	Quality Criteria: Positive Rating
Content validity	A clear description is provided of the measurement aim, the target population, the concepts that are being measured, and the item selection; and target population and investigators and/or experts were involved in item selection
Internal consistency	Factor analyses performed on adequate sample size (7 $\times$ # items and $\geq$100), and Cronbach α calculated per dimension, and Cronbach α between 0.70 and 0.95
Criterion validity	Convincing argument that gold standard is gold, and correlation with gold standard $\geq$0.70
Construct validity	Specific hypotheses were formulated, and at least 75% of the results are in accordance with these hypotheses
Reliability	Intraclass correlation coefficient (for continuous measures) or weighted κ (for ordinal measures) $\geq$0.70
Responsiveness	SDC or SDC < MCID or MCID outside the limits of agreement or Guyatt responsiveness ratio >1.96 or area under the receiver operating curve $\geq$0.70
Floor and ceiling effects	$\leq$15% of the respondents achieved the highest or lowest possible scores
Interpretability	Mean and standard deviation scores presented for at least 4 relevant subgroups of patients, and MCID defined

Abbreviation: SDC, smallest detectable change.
Adapted from Terwee CB, Bot SD, de Boer MR, et al. Quality criteria were proposed for measurement properties of health status questionnaires. J Clin Epidemiol 2007;60:34–42; with permission.

guidelines as to how readers can critically evaluate published results. The Consensus-based Standards for the Selection of Health Measurement Instruments (COSMIN) study group has presented results of a 4-round Delphi study, releasing additional guidelines on evaluating the methodological quality of studies on health status measurement instruments.[45] These guidelines include taxonomy of relationships of measured properties (**Fig. 1**), and a thorough analysis of what properties and methods must be used and reported for the study to be of adequate quality.[41,45] The COSMIN group has challenged some of the traditional tools and methods used in vetting these studies, and developed a series of checklists that guide thorough analysis of published results.[45,46] These sets of standards and checklists are not intended to rate the specific instruments; rather, they provide a systematic approach to evaluating the studies that report on instrument quality, regardless of the study's conclusion.[46] Based on these standards, numerous systematic reviews have assessed the measurement properties and clinimetrics of available PRO metrics.[33,47,48] One such study evaluated the clinimetric properties of instruments used to assess patients with hand

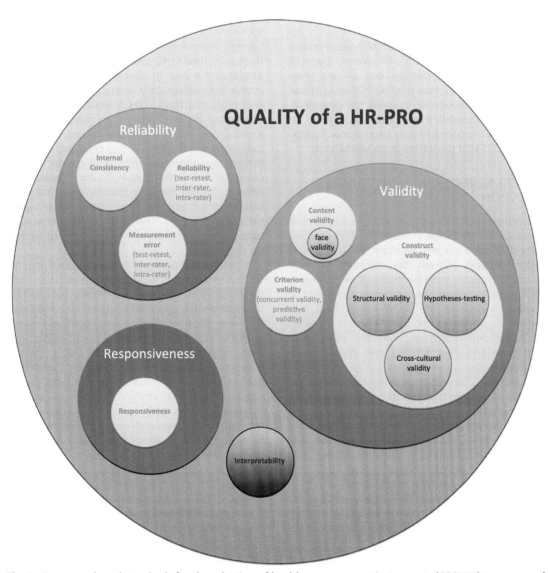

Fig. 1. Consensus-based standards for the selection of health measurement instruments (COSMIN) taxonomy of relationships of measurement properties. HR-PRO, health-related patient-reported outcome. (*From* Mokkink LB, Terwee CB, Patrick DL, et al. The COSMIN study reached international consensus on taxonomy, terminology, and definitions of measurement properties for health-related patient-reported outcomes. J Clin Epidemiol 2010;63:737–45; with permission.)

injuries.[49] They concluded that most functional and patient-reported measures have been inadequately evaluated. MHQ, DASH, and CTQ are 3 of only 5 questionnaires to receive strong ratings, in that well-executed studies properly report reliability, validity, and responsiveness of these metrics.

In addition, the COSMIN group published consensus definitions for the extensive terminology used in determining PRO metric quality.[41] Consistency in the language used to report results improves the value and reliability of primary analyses, systematic reviews, and meta-analyses. The guidelines released by Terwee and colleagues,[44] followed by the COSMIN group's reports, have made great progress toward improving the quality of outcomes measurement. However, these tools are still limited, because use of COSMIN guidelines has shown lower inter-rater reliability than desired.[33] This is in part because of inexperience in using the guidelines, as well as inconsistent use of terminology by the raters. When implemented by experienced investigators, COSMIN guidelines are a useful tool.

PRACTICAL DECISIONS IN INSTRUMENT SELECTION

Using these guidelines and definitions can remove some of the challenge in reviewing this complex subset of hand surgery literature. However, even before looking through the literature, a more practical decision must be made: does the metric to be used contain the proper components to thoroughly evaluate the disease, treatment, and patient population in question? For this there are no developed guidelines, and the investigator must use empirical analysis and questionnaire evaluation.

Consider CTS, which has symptomatic and functional disease manifestations. Understanding that functional metrics do not capture all aspects of the patient's experience and postoperative recovery, the CTQ was designed for use with patients with CTS, and is more responsive than traditional functional metrics.[34] The MHQ and DASH are also responsive instruments for CTS.[24] The pain subdomain of MHQ has a large effect size, and overall MHQ score and DASH score have a moderate effect. Both outperform the SF-36 for CTS.[24,50]

When preparing to do a study on CTS, it is important to consider what each questionnaire can provide. A well-validated disease-specific metric is available; however, this would limit the ability to compare results across other diseases, because the CTQ is not validated for use in most

upper extremity conditions. Using the MHQ or DASH would provide valid outcomes evaluation that could then be further analyzed and even compared with other patient populations for usefulness, cost-effectiveness, or other health-related outcomes.[51] Considering that the MHQ has separate subscales for symptom and functional scores and evaluates the right and left hand separately, the decision is whether these additional elements provide desirable benefits compared with other available questionnaires.

Functional metrics have also traditionally been measured in patients with distal radius fractures. Range of motion and grip strength are important indicators of patient recovery.[52] Unlike with CTS, these measures perform as well as PROs in indicating treatment outcomes after distal radius fracture.[30] The MHQ and DASH have both been validated for use in these patients.[29,30] These instruments adequately evaluate function, ADLs, and pain, and the DASH is highly responsive in the first 3 months after injury when functional metrics are more difficult to evaluate.[29] A third questionnaire, the PRWE, has also been found to have a large effect size and slightly greater responsiveness than the DASH.[29] This instrument, although robust for wrist disorders, has not been validated for use with as many other upper extremity disorders. The questionnaires also evaluate patient satisfaction, which functional metrics do not explore.

In studies on patients with distal radius fractures, the system-specific questionnaires provide additional insight into the domains of pain and satisfaction that are not provided by functional measures. However, the MHQ, DASH, and PRWE all lack the ability to ascertain a greater sense of global well-being and overall health status that a general measure would provide. Adding an additional questionnaire that measures social and mental components of outcomes can give a more comprehensive evaluation of the whole patient experience. RA, with emotional and physical manifestations beyond the upper extremity, is at the opposite end of the spectrum from fractures. General PROs, including SF-36, AIMS2, and the Health Assessment Questionnaire (HAQ), have been validated for RA by numerous studies.[26,27,53,54] These questionnaires have a high responsiveness for patients with RA. In evaluating rheumatoid hand function, a system-specific instrument can also be used. The MHQ is validated in this population, both in those who underwent metacarpophalangeal (MCP) arthroplasty and those who did not have surgical correction of MCP disease.[55] The subdomains and overall scores correlated with aspects of the disease without surgical treatment as well as in postoperative recovery, and showed construct validity compared with AIMS2. Even with these results, when considering the substantial psychosocial overtones of this condition, using any system-specific questionnaire alone for a study on hand function in RA would not capture general health status components of this disease. Therefore, it is important to consider adding a questionnaire that measures the psychosocial component of RA.

MINIMIZING PATIENT BURDEN

When attempting to capture the multidimensional aspects of a complex disease, longer questionnaires are known to have more incomplete data, lower response rates, and often lesser quality results because of responder fatigue and loss to follow-up.[56–58] Several outcomes tools have now been shortened. For example, the SF-36 and the MHQ have been restructured to create the SF12 and the Brief-MHQ.[56,59] These questionnaires use only 1 or 2 items to assess each domain. Although the shortened questionnaire may lose some precision, it can enhance responder compliance by making it less strenuous to complete the questionnaire. These shortened questionnaires have been developed through rigorous methodology, and thus far have performed at or above the level of their more comprehensive predecessors.[59–61]

Another difficulty to consider in upper extremity PRO metric design and use is ceiling and floor effects, in which too many patients score in the highest or lowest range because of inadequate discrimination between patients with different degrees of recovery.[62] With a ceiling effect, some patients with residual impairment are already scoring at the maximum level. A floor effect results in patients having the lowest possible score even when they are in worse condition than others with similar low scores. Upper extremity metrics more often risk ceiling effects.[15] The full-version questionnaires have optimized item quality to minimize a ceiling effect, which is one of the benefits of having the larger number of items. When reducing the number of questions, there is great potential for augmenting a ceiling effect. The ideal is to identify the smallest number of questions that provide precision and also allows for adequately stratifying patients.

To address these issues, investigators have used concepts guided by item response theory (IRT) to design and refine computerized adaptive testing (CAT). IRT uses each item as an indicator of ability or condition, modeling the answer by a respondent with a certain degree of function or ability to each of the items in the questionnaire.[57]

This method provides insight into the responder's abilities or skills based on how they answer each item. With IRT, item number can be decreased, metrics can be standardized, and results can meaningfully be compared; this is also true for questionnaires translated into different languages.[63,64] Although initially used for educational and psychological testing, IRT has also provided unique tools for improving questionnaire design and use in health services research. For example, IRT was used to develop an alternate summary score for the 10-item Physical Functioning (PF-10) scale of the SF-36.[65] The new summative scale had improved precision, especially in patients with scores well above or below median. The use of IRT has subsequently increased rapidly.

IRT has also guided the design and use of CAT, a model in which the instrument progressively adapts to the individual answering the questions.[57] Based on how a question is answered, the next question can be selected and geared to provide more discerning information about the patient's condition. This system allows for the overall question bank to remain large (which helps to minimize ceiling and floor effects) while asking questions that provide adequate stratification of patient conditions and keeping the overall number of questions low.

THE FUTURE OF OUTCOMES MEASUREMENT

Use of IRT-based techniques and the shift toward CAT have changed how health services researchers approach PROs. CAT has been used to improve measurement precision over a wide range of health conditions and has also reduced testing burden.[57] Furthering these efforts, the US National Institutes of Health have focused on developing and using the Patient-Reported Outcomes Measurement Information System (PROMIS).[66] PROMIS includes a growing bank of thoroughly vetted and tested questionnaire items, and divides them into key domains; for example, pain, fatigue, and physical function. Using IRT, different scales and questionnaires have been developed and geared toward specific patient populations, supplanting general PRO questionnaires. These methods have yet to substantially affect hand and upper extremity PRO evaluation. However, the physical function item banks include subsets for upper extremity function.[67,68] In addition, an upper extremity function scale has been created for use with pediatric patients with cancer.[66] Investigators have also shown improved responsiveness with reduction in floor and ceiling effects with IRT-based PROMIS instruments for patients with RA.[69] As these tools are developed and refined, there may be a reduction in the need for disease-specific or symptom-specific metrics.

SUMMARY

In measuring hand surgery outcomes, there are unique challenges. Improving how the physical, emotional, aesthetic, and psychological components of disease are evaluated has resulted in substantial change. Shifting to PROs ushered in the current era of hand surgery–related health services research. However, inconsistent design and use of PRO metrics contributes to continued deficiencies in appropriately measuring outcomes.

It is important to choose the questionnaire(s) that suit study needs. Making assumptions about how the disease affects patients leads to better study design and outcomes tool selection. In addition, the investigator must be careful to avoid overburdening subjects with numerous tests and questionnaires. Finding the right combination of outcomes metrics without compromising study quality can be mitigated in part by thoughtful selection of robust and appropriate instruments. As the use of IRT and CAT continues to mold the future of health services and outcomes research, measuring outcomes in hand surgery will again require a shift in technique, metric design, and study execution. As it becomes increasingly important to make these changes, both for patients and for developing sustainable practice models in an evolving health care climate, improving and maintaining efficiency, quality, and consistency must define hand surgery outcomes research.

REFERENCES

1. Nonfatal occupational injuries and illnesses requiring days away from work, 2010. Bureau of Labor Statistics; 2011. USDL-11-1612.
2. de Putter CE, Selles RW, Polinder S, et al. Economic impact of hand and wrist injuries: health-care costs and productivity costs in a population-based study. J Bone Joint Surg Am 2012;94:e56.
3. Chernew ME, Rosen AB, Fendrick AM. Value-based insurance design. Health Aff (Millwood) 2007;26: w195–203.
4. Choudhry NK, Rosenthal MB, Milstein A. Assessing the evidence for value-based insurance design. Health Aff (Millwood) 2010;29:1988–94.
5. Available at: www.choosingwisely.org.
6. Share DA, Mason MH. Michigan's physician group incentive program offers a regional model for incremental 'fee for value' payment reform. Health Aff (Millwood) 2012;31:1993–2001.
7. Landman JH. Recommendations for delivering value. Healthc Financ Manage 2012;66:98, 100.
8. Epstein AM. The outcomes movement–will it get us where we want to go? N Engl J Med 1990;323: 266–70.
9. Eisenberg JM. Putting research to work: reporting and enhancing the impact of health services research. Health Serv Res 2001;36:x–xvii.
10. Bindra RR, Dias JJ, Heras-Palau C, et al. Assessing outcome after hand surgery: the current state. J Hand Surg Br 2003;28:289–94.
11. Crosby CA, Wehbe MA, Mawr B. Hand strength: normative values. J Hand Surg Am 1994;19:665–70.
12. LaStayo PC, Wheeler DL. Reliability of passive wrist flexion and extension goniometric measurements: a multicenter study. Phys Ther 1994;74:162–74 [discussion: 174–66].
13. Berkanovic E, Hurwicz ML, Lachenbruch PA. Concordant and discrepant views of patients' physical functioning. Arthritis Care Res 1995;8:94–101.
14. Hewlett SA. Patients and clinicians have different perspectives on outcomes in arthritis. J Rheumatol 2003;30:877–9.
15. Szabo RM. Outcomes assessment in hand surgery: when are they meaningful? J Hand Surg Am 2001; 26:993–1002.
16. Alderman AK, Chung KC. Measuring outcomes in hand surgery. Clin Plast Surg 2008;35:239–50.
17. Ware JE Jr. Standards for validating health measures: definition and content. J Chronic Dis 1987; 40:473–80.
18. Zlowodzki M, Bhandari M. Outcome measures and implications for sample-size calculations. J Bone Joint Surg Am 2009;91(Suppl 3):35–40.
19. Changulani M, Okonkwo U, Keswani T, et al. Outcome evaluation measures for wrist and hand: which one to choose? Int Orthop 2008;32:1–6.
20. Davis Sears E, Chung KC. A guide to interpreting a study of patient-reported outcomes. Plast Reconstr Surg 2012;129:1200–7.
21. Fitzpatrick R, Davey C, Buxton MJ, et al. Evaluating patient-based outcome measures for use in clinical trials. Health Technol Assess 1998;2:i–iv, 1–74.
22. Chung KC, Pillsbury MS, Walters MR, et al. Reliability and validity testing of the Michigan Hand Outcomes Questionnaire. J Hand Surg Am 1998; 23:575–87.
23. Beaton DE, Katz JN, Fossel AH, et al. Measuring the whole or the parts? Validity, reliability, and responsiveness of the Disabilities of the Arm, Shoulder and Hand outcome measure in different regions of the upper extremity. J Hand Ther 2001;14:128–46.
24. Kotsis SV, Chung KC. Responsiveness of the Michigan Hand Outcomes Questionnaire and the Disabilities of the Arm, Shoulder and Hand questionnaire in carpal tunnel surgery. J Hand Surg Am 2005;30:81–6.

25. Ware JE Jr, Sherbourne CD. The MOS 36-item short-form health survey (SF-36). I. Conceptual framework and item selection. Med Care 1992;30:473–83.

26. Linde L, Sorensen J, Ostergaard M, et al. Health-related quality of life: validity, reliability, and responsiveness of SF-36, 15D, EQ-5D [corrected] RAQoL, and HAQ in patients with rheumatoid arthritis. J Rheumatol 2008;35:1528–37.

27. Oude Voshaar MA, ten Klooster PM, Taal E, et al. Measurement properties of physical function scales validated for use in patients with rheumatoid arthritis: a systematic review of the literature. Health Qual Life Outcomes 2011;9:99.

28. Aktekin LA, Eser F, Baskan BM, et al. Disability of Arm Shoulder and Hand Questionnaire in rheumatoid arthritis patients: relationship with disease activity, HAQ, SF-36. Rheumatol Int 2011;31:823–6.

29. MacDermid JC, Richards RS, Donner A, et al. Responsiveness of the short form-36, disability of the arm, shoulder, and hand questionnaire, patient-rated wrist evaluation, and physical impairment measurements in evaluating recovery after a distal radius fracture. J Hand Surg Am 2000;25:330–40.

30. Kotsis SV, Lau FH, Chung KC. Responsiveness of the Michigan Hand Outcomes Questionnaire and physical measurements in outcome studies of distal radius fracture treatment. J Hand Surg Am 2007;32:84–90.

31. Chung KC, Burns PB, Davis Sears E. Outcomes research in hand surgery: where have we been and where should we go? J Hand Surg Am 2006;31:1373–9.

32. Meenan RF, Mason JH, Anderson JJ, et al. AIMS2. The content and properties of a revised and expanded Arthritis Impact Measurement Scales Health Status Questionnaire. Arthritis Rheum 1992;35:1–10.

33. Hoang-Kim A, Pegreffi F, Moroni A, et al. Measuring wrist and hand function: common scales and checklists. Injury 2011;42:253–8.

34. Levine DW, Simmons BP, Koris MJ, et al. A self-administered questionnaire for the assessment of severity of symptoms and functional status in carpal tunnel syndrome. J Bone Joint Surg Am 1993;75:1585–92.

35. Beaton DE, Bombardier C, Guillemin F, et al. Guidelines for the process of cross-cultural adaptation of self-report measures. Spine (Phila Pa 1976) 2000;25:3186–91.

36. Gonzalez-Calvo J, Gonzalez VM, Lorig K. Cultural diversity issues in the development of valid and reliable measures of health status. Arthritis Care Res 1997;10:448–56.

37. Van Ommeren M. Validity issues in transcultural epidemiology. Br J Psychiatry 2003;182:376–8.

38. Roh YH, Yang BK, Noh JH, et al. Cross-cultural adaptation and validation of the Korean version of the Michigan hand questionnaire. J Hand Surg Am 2011;36:1497–503.

39. Esposito N. From meaning to meaning: the influence of translation techniques on non-English focus group research. Qual Health Res 2001;11:568–79.

40. Mokkink LB, Terwee CB, Stratford PW, et al. Evaluation of the methodological quality of systematic reviews of health status measurement instruments. Qual Life Res 2009;18:313–33.

41. Mokkink LB, Terwee CB, Patrick DL, et al. The COSMIN study reached international consensus on taxonomy, terminology, and definitions of measurement properties for health-related patient-reported outcomes. J Clin Epidemiol 2010;63:737–45.

42. Jaeschke R, Singer J, Guyatt GH. Measurement of health status. Ascertaining the minimal clinically important difference. Control Clin Trials 1989;10:407–15.

43. Shauver MJ, Chung KC. The minimal clinically important difference of the Michigan hand outcomes questionnaire. J Hand Surg Am 2009;34:509–14.

44. Terwee CB, Bot SD, de Boer MR, et al. Quality criteria were proposed for measurement properties of health status questionnaires. J Clin Epidemiol 2007;60:34–42.

45. Mokkink LB, Terwee CB, Patrick DL, et al. The COSMIN checklist for assessing the methodological quality of studies on measurement properties of health status measurement instruments: an international Delphi study. Qual Life Res 2010;19:539–49.

46. Angst F. The new COSMIN guidelines confront traditional concepts of responsiveness. BMC Med Res Methodol 2011;11:152 [author reply: 152].

47. Oftedal S, Bell KL, Mitchell LE, et al. A systematic review of the clinimetric properties of habitual physical activity measures in young children with a motor disability. Int J Pediatr 2012;2012:976425.

48. Dobson F, Choi YM, Hall M, et al. Clinimetric properties of observer-assessed impairment tests used to evaluate hip and groin impairments: a systematic review. Arthritis Care Res (Hoboken) 2012;64(10):1565–75.

49. van de Ven-Stevens LA, Munneke M, Terwee CB, et al. Clinimetric properties of instruments to assess activities in patients with hand injury: a systematic review of the literature. Arch Phys Med Rehabil 2009;90:151–69.

50. Gay RE, Amadio PC, Johnson JC. Comparative responsiveness of the disabilities of the arm, shoulder, and hand, the carpal tunnel questionnaire, and the SF-36 to clinical change after carpal tunnel release. J Hand Surg Am 2003;28:250–4.

51. Chatterjee JS, Price PE. Comparative responsiveness of the Michigan Hand Outcomes Questionnaire and the Carpal Tunnel Questionnaire after carpal tunnel release. J Hand Surg Am 2009;34:273–80.

52. Chung KC, Haas A. Relationship between patient satisfaction and objective functional outcome after

surgical treatment for distal radius fractures. J Hand Ther 2009;22:302–7 [quiz: 308].

53. Tugwell P, Idzerda L, Wells GA. Generic quality-of-life assessment in rheumatoid arthritis. Am J Manag Care 2008;14:234.

54. Russell AS. Quality-of-life assessment in rheumatoid arthritis. Pharmacoeconomics 2008;26:831–46.

55. Waljee JF, Chung KC, Kim HM, et al. Validity and responsiveness of the Michigan Hand Questionnaire in patients with rheumatoid arthritis: a multicenter, international study. Arthritis Care Res (Hoboken) 2010;62:1569–77.

56. Ware J Jr, Kosinski M, Keller SD. A 12-Item Short-Form Health Survey: construction of scales and preliminary tests of reliability and validity. Med Care 1996;34:220–33.

57. Ware JE Jr. Improvements in short-form measures of health status: introduction to a series. J Clin Epidemiol 2008;61:1–5.

58. Holland R, Smith RD, Harvey I, et al. Assessing quality of life in the elderly: a direct comparison of the EQ-5D and AQoL. Health Econ 2004;13: 793–805.

59. Waljee JF, Kim HM, Burns PB, et al. Development of a brief, 12-item version of the Michigan Hand Questionnaire. Plast Reconstr Surg 2011;128:208–20.

60. Osthus TB, Preljevic VT, Sandvik L, et al. Mortality and health-related quality of life in prevalent dialysis patients: comparison between 12- items and 36-items short-form health survey. Health Qual Life Outcomes 2012;10:46.

61. Gandhi SK, Salmon JW, Zhao SZ, et al. Psychometric evaluation of the 12-item short-form health survey (SF-12) in osteoarthritis and rheumatoid arthritis clinical trials. Clin Ther 2001;23:1080–98.

62. Guyatt GH, Feeny DH, Patrick DL. Measuring health-related quality of life. Ann Intern Med 1993;118: 622–9.

63. Mokkink LB, Knol DL, van Nispen RM, et al. Improving the quality and applicability of the Dutch scales of the Communication Profile for the Hearing Impaired using item response theory. J Speech Lang Hear Res 2010;53:556–71.

64. Jafari P, Bagheri Z, Ayatollahi SM, et al. Using Rasch rating scale model to reassess the psychometric properties of the Persian version of the PedsQL 4.0 Generic Core Scales in school children. Health Qual Life Outcomes 2012;10:27.

65. McHorney CA, Haley SM, Ware JE Jr. Evaluation of the MOS SF-36 Physical Functioning Scale (PF-10): II. Comparison of relative precision using Likert and Rasch scoring methods. J Clin Epidemiol 1997;50:451–61.

66. Available at: www.nihpromis.org.

67. Hung M, Clegg DO, Greene T, et al. Evaluation of the PROMIS physical function item bank in orthopaedic patients. J Orthop Res 2011;29:947–53.

68. DeWitt EM, Stucky BD, Thissen D, et al. Construction of the eight-item patient-reported outcomes measurement information system pediatric physical function scales: built using item response theory. J Clin Epidemiol 2011;64:794–804.

69. Fries J, Rose M, Krishnan E. The PROMIS of better outcome assessment: responsiveness, floor and ceiling effects, and Internet administration. J Rheumatol 2011;38:1759–64.

Measuring Outcomes in Lower Limb Surgery

Adeyiza O. Momoh, MD, Kevin C. Chung, MD, MS*

KEYWORDS

• Outcomes • Lower limb • Salvage • Amputation • Function

KEY POINTS

- Preoperative lower extremity injury scoring systems to aid with surgical decision-making are limited in their ability to clearly predict the need for amputation.
- Patient-reported outcomes after limb salvage and amputation play a critical role in assessing the quality and efficacy of surgical strategies used.
- Patients with severe lower extremity injuries have significant levels of disability following limb salvage and amputations.
- Limb salvage procedures are successful but are associated with higher rates of complication than amputations.
- Long-term functional outcomes are similar in patients with salvaged and amputated lower extremities, with no difference in their ability to return to work.
- Level of amputation does not affect a patient's perceptions of their results.
- The absence of plantar sensation at initial presentation is not a predictor of the need to amputate.
- Delays in the initial wound debridement beyond 24 hours are associated with higher rates of amputation.
- Self-efficacy is one of the strongest predictors of a patient's ability to return to work.
- Postoperative self-management interventions have the potential to improve overall function and quality of life in these patients.
- Satisfaction is not influenced by treatment strategy but by postoperative function, pain, and the presence or absence of depression.
- Limb salvage has a higher utility value and costs less than amputation.
- Results from studies in the trauma population are not generalizable to other patient groups.

INTRODUCTION

Limb salvage requires persistent effort for patients with aggressive lower extremity tumors or severe peripheral vascular disease with tissue loss, and in patients who have sustained traumatic complex lower extremity injuries. Important reconstructive considerations in all patients regardless of the cause of their limb disease are limb vascularity, tissue components involved that require replacement or stabilization, and the potential for restoration of function with limb salvage. Our ability to

Supported in part by grants from the National Institute on Aging and National Institute of Arthritis and Musculoskeletal and Skin Diseases (R01 AR062066) and from the National Institute of Arthritis and Musculoskeletal and Skin Diseases (2R01 AR047328-06) and a Midcareer Investigator Award in Patient-Oriented Research (K24 AR053120) (to Dr Kevin C. Chung).
Section of Plastic Surgery, The University of Michigan Medical School, 2130 Taubman Center, SPC 5340, 1500 East Medical Center Drive, Ann Arbor, MI 48109-5340, USA
* Corresponding author.
E-mail address: kecchung@umich.edu

salvage the severely injured lower extremity has improved with technical advances[1,2] over the years. As would be expected, the question of whether salvage is beneficial to certain patients with severe injuries has been raised and some[3,4] have justifiably suggested that early amputation and rehabilitation with prosthesis provide a better outcome in select patients. In contrast, others[5] have found that most of their patients with severe lower extremity injuries preferred their salvaged extremity to an amputation, even when they ultimately required a delayed amputation. Although appealing, limb salvage may not always be in the best interest of patients because limb viability and function do not always go hand in hand.

Given that the decision to amputate or salvage an extremity is one of the first decisions made in managing patients with severe lower extremity injuries, preoperative scoring systems to aid with the decision-making process would be useful and have been developed.[6–9] However, the utility of existing scoring systems has been called into question, because they have been found to be effective at identifying patients who would benefit from salvage but are incapable of identifying patients who would ultimately require amputation.[10] This incapability is a significant flaw because amputations performed in a timely fashion can potentially provide patients with a shorter recovery and return to a relatively high level of function with the use of prostheses. Without a clear consensus on preoperative findings that guide decisions, surgeons in practice have to make decisions based on their clinical judgment, sometimes with little or no supporting evidence.

An understanding of outcomes after salvage is also critical to guiding the surgical decision-making process when considering the choice of limb salvage versus amputation. Surgical outcomes focused on complications and function from the physician's viewpoint provide valuable information but do not provide a complete picture. To this end, as in other areas of health care, considerations of patient-reported outcomes have become an integral part of assessing the quality and efficacy of care delivered. The term patient-reported outcomes broadly includes functional assessments and health-related quality-of-life outcomes. Outcomes are assessed from the patient's viewpoint and they have the potential to be distinctly different from those perceived by the treating physician. These outcomes ideally should provide some clarity to questions, such as: Is it more beneficial to salvage or amputate an extremity? Which patients would benefit from limb salvage as opposed to an amputation? Does the level of injury make a difference? Are there surgical or patient factors outside of the injury that have an impact on a patient's ultimate function and quality of life? Are there injury-related factors that have an impact on patient-reported outcomes? How satisfied are patients postoperatively? and What are the financial implications of these treatment strategies?

PATIENT-REPORTED OUTCOMES MEASURES

Patient-reported outcomes measures (PROMs) are obtained by way of patient-completed questionnaires that assess a host of health-related outcomes relating to patient function and quality of life after undergoing surgery. In general, these outcomes measures can be used to evaluate the quality of care delivered, to assess the efficacy and cost-effectiveness of multiple treatment modalities, and to guide patient choice. Findings from these instruments allow surgeons to better understand salient aspects of a patient's experience after major limb operations, including but not limited to their ability to walk, care for themselves, work, and participate in recreational activities, as well as the effect of these operations on social interactions and sexual function. Ultimately, information gathered based on patient-rated outcomes can be used to improve surgical management choices in patients with significant lower extremity injuries. Functional assessments are a key component of health and well-being in the lower extremity trauma patient. Self-reported measures rely on a patient's perception of mobility status and performance of activities of daily living. These measures aim to assess a patient's activity restrictions, performance difficulties, or the need for assistance with functional activities.

Health-related quality-of-life outcomes are the other component of well-being measured by PROMs. This outcomes measure essentially is an assessment of what health status is worth to a patient, from the patient's perspective after an injury or intervention. Generic measurement instruments cover areas of relevance to multiple disorders and are applicable to the general population to compare among different groups. Specific instruments, in contrast, are tailored to particular disease processes. As PROMs present data solely from the patient's perspective, patient factors such as poor cognitive function, culture, language, and education can have an influence on outcomes reported.

Multiple questionnaires for lower extremity outcomes have been developed (**Table 1**), with the more commonly used questionnaires in recent years including the Sickness Impact Profile (SIP),[11] the Toronto Extremity Salvage Score,[12]

Table 1
Selected measurement instruments

Instrument	Measure	Scoring	Primary Outcomes Evaluated
The Sickness Impact Profile (SIP)	Generic, behaviorally based, health status measure	Scores range from 0 to 100; scores >10 represent severe disability	Health-related dysfunction in 12 categories—ambulation, mobility, body care and movement, social interaction, alertness, emotional behavior, communication, sleep and rest, eating, work, home management, and recreation
Musculo-Skeletal Tumor Society (MSTS)	Disease-specific instrument (musculoskeletal tumors)	Scores range from 0 to 30; value of 0 to 5 is assigned to each of 6 categories. Higher scores indicate better function	Pain, function, emotional acceptance, supports, walking, and gait
Toronto Extremity Salvage Score (TESS)	Disease-specific instrument (extremity sarcoma)	Scores range from 0 to 100; 30 items are rated on a 5-point Likert scale	Activity limitations, restrictions in mobility, restrictions in self care, and restrictions in performing daily tasks and routines
Nottingham Health Profile (NHP)	Generic health status measure	Scores range from 0 to 100; higher numbers indicate greater disability	Part I: Subjective health status—mobility, energy level, pain, sleep, emotional reactions, social isolation. Part II: Influence of health problems on—employment, housework, family life, social life, sexual function, recreation, and enjoyment of holidays
Short Form (36) Health Survey (SF-36)	Generic health-related quality of life measure	Scores range from 0 to 100; higher numbers indicate a better health state	8 scales assessed resulting in scores relating to patients' perceived physical and mental status—vitality, physical functioning, bodily pain, general health perceptions, physical role functioning, emotional role functioning, social role functioning, mental health
Western Ontario and McMaster University Osteoarthritis Index (WOMAC)	Disease specific (arthritis)	Scores range from 0 to 96; higher numbers indicate greater disability	24 items in 3 dimensions—stiffness, pain, and physical function

and the Musculoskeletal Tumor Society Score.[13] The SIP has been used the most in recent studies on lower extremity trauma, whereas instruments such as the Toronto Extremity Salvage Score and Musculoskeletal Tumor Society Score questionnaires were developed specifically for oncologic patients. Generic questionnaires also used in lower extremity trauma studies include the Short Form-36[14] and the Nottingham Health Profile.

REVIEW OF THE RECENT LITERATURE

Most of the data relating to PROMs in patients undergoing limb salvage or amputations are presented in the orthopedic and trauma literature. A basic question in dealing with severe lower extremity injuries is, how do patients fare with amputations relative to salvage? As part of the Lower Extremity Assessment Project (LEAP), Bosse and colleagues[15] analyzed the long-term functional outcomes of salvage when compared to amputation in 545 patients with injuries below the femur. They used the SIP, a multidimensional measure of self-reported health status for functional assessment, to provide information ranging from ambulation and body care to social interactions. At 2 years, no significant difference in scores was found between amputated and reconstructed patients. Patients in both treatment arms on average had significant levels of disability when compared to the general population based on the SIP. Similar proportions of patients from both groups had returned to work at 2 years, although reconstructed patients had significantly higher rates of rehospitalization and reoperation compared to patients with amputations. A problem with this study was the relatively short follow-up, because at 2 years most of the patients are still recovering and improved function may be anticipated with greater periods of time allowed for recovery. Interestingly, a 7-year follow-up on the same cohort of patients actually found a slight deterioration in function in both groups.[16] This deterioration in function was thought to be partly from aging of the cohort with the associated worsening of function that occurs with advancing age. Here again there were no significant differences in the outcomes reported by patients with salvaged or amputated limbs.

Amputations in these studies varied from above the knee proximally to partial foot amputations distally. With an understanding that longer lower extremity lengths in amputees are generally associated with better ambulatory function,[17] it would be reasonable to expect that varying levels of amputations or salvage may have an impact on patient-reported outcomes. Mackenzie and colleagues[18] reported similar SIP scores in patients with above-the-knee amputations compared to patients with amputations below the knee, but injuries in these patients did not involve the foot and ankle. A look at mangled foot and ankle injuries[19] found worse SIP outcomes at 2 years in patients requiring free flaps and ankle fusion when compared to patients who had below the knee amputations. Salvage with simple skin coverage (non-free flap), however, had better results than below the knee amputations. A suggestion was made that the addition of a free flap or an arthrodesis reversed the beneficial effect of salvage; viewed from an alternate perspective, it would seem that the need for a free flap/arthrodesis signifies an injury of greater complexity and as such the poorer outcomes seen in these patients may be a reflection of this level of complexity.

With the data for these outcomes coming from the patient, patient-related factors may have a significant impact on the findings reported. A few studies[15,20–22] have reported on a relationship between self-efficacy and social support on outcomes. From the LEAP study,[23] self-efficacy was one of the strongest predictors of return to work. Self-efficacy has to do with a patient's confidence in their ability to perform a specific task or activity. Patients with low self-efficacy expect to fail at specific tasks and as a result they tend to disengage from the coping process. These findings support the need for interventions in the early phase of recovery to address the psychosocial needs of patients, assisting them with self-managing the multifactorial consequences of their injury. There is some evidence in the treatment of other disorders[24,25] that self-management interventions based on cognitive-behavioral theory increase self-efficacy, decreasing secondary conditions such as anxiety, pain, and depression; overall improvements in function and quality of life are also reported. Other patient characteristics associated with poor outcomes include older age, female sex, nonwhite race, lower level of education, living in a poor household, a current or previous history of smoking, poor self-reported preinjury health status, and an involvement with the legal system for obtaining disability payments.[15,16] Unfortunately many of these factors are overrepresented in the severe lower extremity trauma population. Nevertheless, these patients have preferences with regard to their treatment options even though a good portion of them are unable to make these decisions at presentation. A recent Web-based survey of patients and physicians used to generate quality-adjusted life-years found that both groups placed a higher value on limb salvage compared to amputations.[26]

Based on the gain in value assigned, patients seem to value limb salvage to an even greater extent than do physicians.

With the goal of getting a better handle on the contribution of multiple injury-related factors to surgical management and outcomes, lower extremity injury severity scoring systems have been developed. These scoring systems attempt to quantify the severity of trauma, assigning numerical values to various aspects of injuries, including patient age, bone, soft tissue, nerve and vascular injury, warm ischemia time, contamination, and the presence of systemic shock. These factors are weighted differently based on their perceived importance in predicting ultimate outcomes. The initial presenting neurologic examination is one such factor that is heavily weighted in scoring systems like the NISSSA (Nerve Injury, Ischemia, Soft-Tissue Injury, Skeletal Injury, Shock, and Age of Patient Score) and HFS-97 (Hannover Fracture Scale-97). Traditionally, even outside of the scoring systems, a critical factor in the decision to amputate has hinged on the absence of plantar sensation that was supported by a retrospective look at factors influencing the decision to amputate or reconstruct limbs after high-energy traumatic injuries.[27] The presence of soft tissue injury and the absence of plantar sensation were 2 of the more important factors in the decision-making process. An investigation on long-term outcomes in the salvage of extremities with absent plantar sensation compared 26 insensate plantar feet that were amputated to 29 insensate plantar feet that were salvaged and 29 matched controls of sensate limbs that were salvaged.[28] Interestingly, at 2 years, equal proportions of patients had normal plantar sensation in the insensate salvaged group and the sensate salvaged group. SIP scores in all groups were similar. The absence of plantar sensation at the time of initial presentation was not predictive of eventual functional outcome or plantar sensation. Plantar sensation did not prove to be an indication for amputation and this is likely explained by the fact that initial presenting nerve dysfunction could be the result of reversible ischemia or neurapraxia as opposed to complete nerve disruption.

The timing of the first operative procedure is a variable of patient management many times in the control of the surgeon. Multiple studies[29–31] have found no association between delays beyond 6 to 8 hours and morbidities such as infections and nonunions. However, an analysis of data from the Nationwide Inpatient Sample by Sears and colleagues[32] found that delays in the first operative procedure beyond 24 hours significantly increased the likelihood of amputations in patients with severe open tibia fractures. This finding held true when controlling for biases introduced by concomitant traumatic injuries that may prevent a timely initial debridement.

In the current health care climate, patient satisfaction has become a key surrogate for assessing quality of care. Unfortunately, little research has been conducted on patient satisfaction with the management of high-energy lower extremity trauma. A retrospective study evaluating patient satisfaction was conducted on a series of 148 patients who had amputations ranging from the hip to the transmetatarsal level.[33] Patient-perceived results did not correlate with the level of amputations but rather were found to be related to the function of prostheses used and the patient's ability to manage social activities and interactions. The results of this study, although important, are of limited use in considering amputations or limb salvage for trauma because patients in the study had amputations for a variety of other reasons, including infections, congenital defects, vascular disease, diabetes, and tumors. Additionally, because only patients with amputations were studied, information on satisfaction in patients with salvaged extremities is not available. More recently, O'Toole and colleagues[34] investigated patient satisfaction in the severe lower extremity injury patient population, comparing amputated and limb salvage patients. Patient demographic data, treatment type, or specific injury characteristics did not correlate with satisfaction. Five outcomes measures accounted for over one-third of the variations seen in patient satisfaction—return to work, depression, physical function as measured by the SIP, self-selected walking speed, and pain intensity. Based on this study, it would seem that neither of the surgical treatments (amputation or limb salvage) affects the level of satisfaction reported by patients but rather function, pain, and the presence or absence of depression play significant roles.

Given the limited available resources for health care and the similarities in outcomes for both treatment strategies, the financial implications of managing these patients are important considerations in the decision-making process. Using data from the LEAP study, Chung and colleagues[35] performed a cost-utility analysis of amputations and limb salvage in patients with the most severe open tibial fractures. Amputations were found to be more expensive than limb salvage, independent of the costs for prosthesis needs. Salvage was also found to have a higher utility than amputation, and these differences were amplified in younger patients. In the absence of clear indications for an amputation, salvage should be a strong consideration based on reasons of cost-effectiveness and higher utility from the patient's perspective.

LIMITATIONS OF STUDIES/OUTCOMES INSTRUMENTS

As is the case with much of the surgical literature, based on the nature of injuries and conditions being treated, most of the studies looking at functional and quality-of-life outcomes with amputations and limb salvage did not randomize patients into treatment arms. Clinical decisions were made regarding surgical treatment at the time of initial presentation, and outcomes were investigated after the fact. Typically, patients with more severe injuries end up with amputations as opposed to salvage. This selection bias inherent in these studies could have influenced some of the results reported.

The outcomes observed in most of these studies are specific to severe high-energy traumatic injuries and are not generalizable to other patient populations, such as patients who sustain injuries in military conflicts and oncologic patients. The nature of the injuries, as well as unique external patient factors that contribute to the ultimate outcomes, further prevents generalization of the results.

Unfortunately, the information available from patient-reported outcomes does not help predict which limbs should be salvaged and which should be amputated in the trauma population.

SUMMARY

Ideal scoring systems that aid with the decision on limb salvage versus amputation are lacking. Assessing postoperative functional and health-related quality-of-life outcomes with a variety of patient-reported measures are a way of better understanding some of the nuances associated with amputations or limb salvage. The data from the literature suggest similar functional outcomes and rates of return to work in patients with salvaged and amputated lower extremities, although salvage procedures are plagued by higher rates of complication and reoperation. Multiple patient factors associated with poor outcomes cannot be changed; however, strategies to improve on self-efficacy can potentially improve on outcomes in both groups of patients and early debridements may decrease the need for amputations. Limb salvage provides cost-savings and seems to have a greater utility value to patients relative to amputations. More work will need to be done to help surgeons to predict consistently and

reliably which patients presenting with severe lower extremity injuries will benefit from limb salvage or an early amputation.

REFERENCES

1. Godina M. Early microsurgical reconstruction of complex trauma of the extremities. Plast Reconstr Surg 1986;78:285–92.
2. Francel TJ, Vander Kolk CA, Hoopes JE, et al. Microvascular soft-tissue transplantation for reconstruction of acute open tibial fractures: timing of coverage and long-term functional results. Plast Reconstr Surg 1992;89:478–87.
3. Hansen ST Jr. The type-IIIC tibial fracture: salvage or amputation. J Bone Joint Surg Am 1987;69:799–800.
4. Georgiadis GM, Behrens FF, Joyce MJ, et al. Open tibial fractures with severe soft-tissue loss: limb salvage compared with below-the-knee amputation. J Bone Joint Surg Am 1993;75:1431–41.
5. Dagum AB, Best AK, Schemitsch EH, et al. Salvage after severe lower-extremity trauma: are the outcomes worth the means? Plast Reconstr Surg 1999;103:1212–20.
6. Howe HR Jr, Poole GV, Hansen KJ, et al. Salvage of lower extremities following combined orthopaedic and vascular trauma: a predictive salvage index. Am Surg 1987;53:205–8.
7. Helfet DL, Howey T, Sanders R, et al. Limb salvage versus amputation: preliminary results of mangled extremity severity score. Clin Orthop 1990;256:80–6.
8. Johansen K, Daines M, Howey T, et al. Objective criteria accurately predict amputation following extremity trauma. J Trauma 1990;30:568–73.
9. Russell WL, Sailors DM, Whittle TB, et al. Limb salvage versus traumatic amputation: a decision based on a seven-part predictive index. Ann Surg 1991;213:473–81.
10. Bosse MJ, Mackenzie EJ, Kellam JF, et al. A prospective evaluation of the clinical utility of the lower-extremity injury-severity scores. J Bone Joint Surg Am 2001;83:3–14.
11. Bergner M, Bobbitt RA, Carter WB, et al. The sickness impact profile: development and final revision of a health status measure. Med Care 1981;19:787–805.
12. Davis AM, Wright JG, Williams JI, et al. Development of a measure of physical function for patients with bone and soft tissue sarcoma. Qual Life Res 1996; 5:508–16.
13. Simon MA, Aschliman MA, Thomas N, et al. Limb salvage treatment versus amputation for osteosarcoma of the distal end of the femur. J Bone Joint Surg Am 1986;68:1331–7.
14. McHorney CA, Ware JE Jr, Raczek AE. The MOS 36-Item short form health survey (SF-36): II. Psychometric and clinical tests of validity in measuring

physical and mental health constructs. Med Care 1993;31:247.

15. Bosse MJ, MacKenzie EJ, Kellam JF, et al. An analysis of outcomes of reconstruction of amputation after leg-threatening injuries. N Engl J Med 2002; 347(24):1924–31.

16. MacKenzie EJ, Bosse MJ, Pollak AN, et al. Long-term persistence of disability following severe lower-limb trauma. Results of a seven-year follow-up. J Bone Joint Surg Am 2005;87(8):1801–9.

17. Penn-Barwell JG. Outcomes in lower limb amputation following trauma: a systematic review and meta-analysis. Injury 2011;42:1474–9.

18. Mackenzie EJ, Bosse MJ, Castillo RC, et al. Functional outcomes following trauma-related lower extremity amputation. J Bone Joint Surg Am 2004; 86(8):1636–45.

19. Ellington JK, Bosse MJ, Castillo RC, et al. The mangled foot and ankle: results from a 2-year prospective study. J Orthop Trauma 2012 [Eup ahead of print].

20. Mock C, MacKenzie E, Jurkovich G, et al. Determinants of disability following lower extremity fracture. J Trauma 2000;49:1002–11.

21. MacKenzie EJ, Morris JA Jr, Jurkovich GJ, et al. Return to work following injury: the role of economic, social, and job-related factors. Am J Public Health 1998;88:1630–7.

22. Kempen G, Scaf-Klomp W, Ranchor A, et al. Social predictors of recovery in late middle-aged and older persons after injury to the extremities: a prospective study. J Gerontol B Psychol Sci Soc Sci 2001;56: S229–36.

23. Mackenzie EJ, Bosse M. Factors influencing outcome following limb-threatening lower limb trauma: lessons learned from the Lower Extremity Assessment Project (LEAP). J Am Acad Orthop Surg 2006;14(10 Spec No):S205–10.

24. Lorig K, Holman H. Arthritis self-management studies: a twelve-year review. Health Educ Q 1993;20:17–28.

25. Lorig KR, Hooman HR. Self management education: history, definition, outcomes and mechanisms. Ann Behav Med 2003;26:1–7.

26. Chung KC, Shauver MJ, Saddawi-Konefka D, et al. A decision analysis of amputation versus reconstruction for severe open tibial fracture from the physician and patient perspectives. Ann Plast Surg 2011;66(2):185–91.

27. MacKenzie EJ, Bosse MJ, Kellam JF, et al. Factors influencing the decision to amputate or reconstruct after high-energy lower extremity trauma. J Trauma 2002;52(4):641–9.

28. Bosse M, McCarthy ML, Jones AL, et al. The insensate foot following severe lower extremity trauma: an indication for amputation? J Bone Joint Surg Am 2005;87(12):2601–8.

29. Skaggs DL, Friend L, Alman B, et al. The effect of surgical delay on acute infection following 554 open fractures in children. J Bone Joint Surg Am 2005;87:8–12.

30. Spencer J, Smith A, Woods D. The effect of time delay on infection in open long-bone fractures: a 5-year prospective audit from a district general hospital. Ann R Coll Surg Engl 2004;86:108–12.

31. Webb LX, Bosse MJ, Castillo RC, et al, LEAP Study Group. Analysis of surgeon-controlled variables in the treatment of limb-threatening type-III open tibial diaphyseal fractures. J Bone Joint Surg Am 2007; 89:923–8.

32. Sears ED, Davis MM, Chung KC. Relationship between timing of emergency procedures and limb amputation in patients with open tibia fracture in the United States, 2003 to 2009. Plast Reconstr Surg 2012;130(2):369–78.

33. Matsen SL, Malchow D, Matsen FA 3rd. Correlations with patients' perspectives of the result of lower-extremity amputation. J Bone Joint Surg Am 2000; 82:1089–95.

34. O'toole R, Castillo R, Pollak A, et al. Determinants of patient satisfaction after severe lower extremity injuries. J Bone Joint Surg Am 2008;90(6): 1206–11.

35. Chung KC, Saddawi-Konefka D, Haase SC, et al. A cost-utility analysis of amputation versus salvage for Gustilo type IIIB and IIIC open tibial fractures. Plast Reconstr Surg 2009;124(6):1965–73.

Measuring Outcomes in Breast Surgery

Valerie Lemaine, MD, MPH, FRCSC[a],
Colleen McCarthy, MD, MS, FRCSC[b],*

KEYWORDS

- Breast reconstruction • Augmentation mammoplasty • Breast reduction • Mastopexy
- Patient-reported outcomes • NSQIP • Morbidity • BREAST-Q

KEY POINTS

- Clinician-reported rating scales used to assess cosmetic outcomes after breast surgery usually demonstrate poor to moderate inter-rater reliability, regardless of the type of scale used to assess the outcome.
- Although the validity of the Baker classification system for capsular contracture severity has been demonstrated, its reliability remains unknown.
- A scoring system designed to assess the severity of breast skin injury after mastectomy and post-mastectomy reconstruction is now available: the Mastectomy SKIN Score.
- Further research is needed to evaluate the measurement tools used to assess donor site morbidity after breast reconstructive surgery.
- The BREAST-Q is a well-developed, validated, breast surgery–specific, patient-reported outcome (PRO) measure that can be used to evaluate patients' perception of outcome after breast reduction, augmentation, or reconstruction.
- The American College of Surgeons National Surgical Quality Improvement Project (NSQIP) is a national outcomes database that can be used to evaluate surgical outcomes after tissue flaps, breast reductions, and breast reconstruction.

INTRODUCTION

In recent years, increased emphasis has been placed on measuring clinical outcomes and improving quality of care in the United States. As a result, a growing number of outcomes-based measures have been developed to assist providers and health care organizations in measuring their performance. This review article provides a summary of the available tools to help surgeons and hospitals achieve measurable improvements in

1. Patient satisfaction after plastic surgery of the breast (ie, breast reduction, augmentation, and reconstruction)
2. Overall quality of care for breast surgical patients

CLINICIAN-REPORTED OUTCOMES

Before the recent advances in PRO measurement, clinician-reported outcome (ClinRO) tools constituted the basis of outcomes assessments in plastic surgery. ClinROs are successfully used to

Funding Sources: Dr McCarthy: Nil. Dr Lemaine: Allergan.
Conflict of Interest: Nil.
[a] Division of Plastic Surgery, Department of Surgery, Mayo Clinic, 200 First Street Southwest, Rochester, MN 55905, USA; [b] Department of Surgery, Memorial Sloan-Kettering Cancer Center, 1275 York Avenue, New York, NY 10065, USA
* Corresponding author.
E-mail address: McCarthC@mskcc.org

Clin Plastic Surg 40 (2013) 331–339
http://dx.doi.org/10.1016/j.cps.2012.12.003

report endpoints that cannot be directly reported by a patient. The main drawback of using a ClinRO tool in plastic surgery is that although a given tool may reliably measure a particular outcome through the eyes of the assessor, it typically does not measure how a patient perceives this outcome. In the setting of breast surgery, this is especially important because surgery is directed toward a restoration or improvement in breast form as realized by the patient. Furthermore, existing data suggest that there may be considerable interobserver variability not only among providers but also between providers and patients when measuring subjective parameters.[1] For instance, in the oncologic literature, several reports have demonstrated some discordance between what providers measure and what patients consider important when assessing toxicity symptoms of cancer treatments.[2–4] In breast surgery, such differences must be recognized by the surgeon preoperatively to set realistic patient expectations and maximize postoperative satisfaction. To that effect, ClinRO tools, when used in combination with validated PRO instruments, still play a role in measuring provider-patient discordance when assessing subjective outcomes after breast surgery.

Cosmetic Outcome After Breast Surgery

The evaluation of aesthetic outcome after breast surgery is by nature a highly subjective process. A literature review identified 2 scales used frequently in recent studies for breast cosmetic assessment by the provider:

1. Harvard scale[1,5]
2. ABNSW scoring system,[6,7] supported by the Japanese Breast Cancer Society

The Harvard scale is a simple ordinal scale consisting of 4 categories: excellent, good, fair, and poor. Four-point scales evaluating the results of breast reconstruction tend to have unacceptable inter-rater reliability because raters use subjective guidelines to characterize each given category.[8]

The ABNSW scoring system contains 5 subscales:

A, Asymmetry
B, Breast shape
N, Nipple deformation
S, Skin condition
W, Wound scar

For each category, a score from 0 to 3 is established as follows:

3: Excellent—both breasts have a similar appearance

2: Good—there are a few differences between both breasts but only on close observation
1: Fair—there are marked differences between the breasts from a distance
0: Poor—there are severe, unattractive differences between the breasts

A total score is then calculated based on the 5 items, where the cosmetic outcome is deemed "Excellent" when the total score is 15 points, "Good" when the total score is between 11 and 14, "Fair" when it is between 6 and 10, and "Poor" when it is less than 6. This type of scale tends to have higher inter-rater reliability because raters follow specific guidelines to characterize each given category, and there is less subjective interpretation.

Reliability of outcome results

When using such instruments, demonstration of the reliability of the results, with acceptable intra-rater and inter-rater reliability, is essential because cosmetic assessments may vary depending on the evaluator or the timing of the assessment.[8] Intra-rater reliability can be calculated using the kappa statistic, which gives the reader a quantitative measure of the magnitude of agreement between raters. Values of the kappa statistic range from −1 (complete disagreement) to +1 (perfect agreement), with a value of 0 representing exactly what is expected by chance. Kappa statistic values are interpreted as follows[8–10]:

- Less than 0.40, poor agreement beyond chance
- 0.40 to 0.75, Fair to good agreement
- Greater than 0.75, excellent agreement above chance

In a recent study by Leonardi and colleagues,[1] the investigators evaluated the impact of medical specialty and provider gender on aesthetic evaluation after autologous breast reconstruction with and without radiation therapy. Raters used the Harvard scale and a numeric scale from 0 (worst result) to 10 (best result) for evaluation of cosmetic outcomes. Overall, there was moderate inter-rater reliability and significant differences among specialties when using a binary classification system of positive/negative judgment. Plastic surgeons' opinions had the most reliable level of agreement ($\kappa = 0.60$ vs $\kappa = 0.45$ and $\kappa = 0.48$ for radiation oncologists and breast surgeons, respectively). Female breast surgeons consistently gave the lowest scores, followed by female radiation oncologists. Regardless of gender, plastic surgeons gave the most uniform opinion and the most favorable aesthetic scores. The analysis using the Harvard scale provided poor to fair inter-rater reliability. Other studies evaluating cosmetic ClinROs after breast reconstruction usually demonstrate poor to moderate inter-rater reliability, regardless of the type of scale used to assess the outcome.[11]

Capsular Contracture

The Baker classification system is the most commonly used and widely accepted rating scale used to grade the severity of implant capsular contracture in the setting of both cosmetic breast augmentation and postmastectomy implant-based reconstruction.[12] This rating scale, a ClinRO instrument, uses clinical examination to guide the assessment of the degree of firmness ± distortion around an implant.

Although the Baker system was originally developed to evaluate capsule formation in the setting of augmentation mammaplasty, modification of the classification system was subsequently applied to better classify capsule formation in the setting of prosthetic breast reconstruction. More specifically, the distinction between the 2 systems was highlighted to address that a significant proportion of reconstructed breasts have what is considered a detectable implant, due not necessarily to capsular contracture but rather to the lack of overlying soft tissue.

For example, in the setting of augmentation mammaplasty:

1. Class I represents a natural looking breast in which the implant is not detectable.

2. Class II assumes some degree of capsular contracture in the augmented breast because the implant is detectable.

In the setting of implant-based reconstruction, class I is subdivided into 2 subgroups: class IA represents a natural looking breast in which the implant is not visible; class IB describes a soft but visible implant secondary to the performance of the mastectomy. By contrast, class II in the modified system represents an implant with mild firmness. In both systems, a class IV contracture represents a symptomatic breast that is excessively firm to the touch and as such is believed to require surgical intervention (**Table 1**).

Although both classification systems are straightforward and easy to use, neither of these systems have undergone formal evaluation that may be applied to rating scales. For example, a literature review reveals that there are no published studies that formally evaluate the Baker classification system for reliability (ie, the extent to which it gives consistent results) or responsiveness to change. Furthermore, concern exists that because the measurement of capsular contracture severity is based on a provider's subjective observation, it may be imprecise and vulnerable to provider/observer bias.

There is evidence, however, which supports the validity of the scale or the degree to which it measures what it is supposed to measure. For example, Zahavi and colleagues[13] compared the clinical assessment of capsular contractures to a radiologic thickness of the capsule, as evaluated

Table 1
Baker classification systems

Original Baker Classification of Capsular Contracture After Augmentation Mammaplasty	
Class I	Breast absolutely natural; no one could tell breast was augmented.
Class II	Minimal contracture; surgeon can tell surgery was performed but patient has not complaint.
Class III	Moderate contracture; patient feels some firmness.
Class IV	Severe contracture; obvious just from observation.
Classification of Capsular Contracture After Prosthetic Breast Reconstruction	
Class IA	Absolutely natural, cannot tell breast was reconstructed.
Class IB	Soft, but the implant is detectable by physical examination or inspection because of mastectomy.
Class II	Mildly firm reconstructed breast with an implant that may be visible and detectable by physical examination.
Class III	Moderately firm reconstructed breast. The implant is readily detectable, but the result may still be acceptable.
Class IV	Severe contracture with an unacceptable aesthetic outcome and/or significant patient symptoms requiring surgical intervention.

by both ultrasound (US) and MRI. A total of 20 patients, with 27 implants, was evaluated in the study. A positive correlation was found between capsular thicknesses as evaluated by either US or MRI and the clinical Baker score, with P values of 0.002 and 0.017, respectively. More specifically, a Baker score of I or II had a thinner capsule, averaging 1.14 mm compared with a Baker score of III or IV, which averaged 2.39 mm. The same correlation was found with MRI, where a Baker score of I or II correlated with a capsule measuring 1.39-mm thick, compared with a Baker score of III or IV, which correlated with a thicker capsule averaging 2.62 mm.

A similar study was undertaken to investigate long-term histologic changes in the environment of breast implants and their correlation at the time of capsular contracture defined by the Baker score.[14] The collagenous capsules of 53 silicone breast implants from 43 patients were evaluated histologically for capsular thickness. A significantly higher degree of the Baker score was found with increasing capsular thickness ($P<.009$).

Although these latter methods of capsular contracture evaluation may provide more objective measurements, they are neither cost effective nor appropriate for routine evaluation of capsule development. There have been several attempts to objectively measure capsular contracture with instruments designed to measure deformability, using tools such as compression clippers or tonometry.[15–17] These methods, which may allow for a more precise measurement tool, may be less valid, because the overlying skin and subcutaneous tissue ± surrounding breast must also be compressed by the instrument, which adds a confounding variable. Thus, in spite of its limitations, the Baker classification system remains the gold standard approach to capsular contracture severity grading at the present time.

Breast Skin Ischemic Injury

With increasing adoption of immediate breast reconstruction (IBR) after skin-sparing mastectomy (SSM) and nipple-sparing mastectomy (NSM), breast skin ischemic injury is a frequently encountered complication. Mastectomy skin necrosis—an umbrella term commonly (and sometimes erroneously) used in the scientific literature to describe a spectrum of postoperative breast skin ischemic injuries—has been the focus of many recent publications.[18–23] Breast skin ischemic injury after mastectomy and IBR may be associated with profound consequences secondary to the breakdown of the skin barrier: it may postpone the initiation of adjuvant therapy

due to delayed wound healing and potentially lead to reoperation for prosthetic infection and reconstruction failure. The incidence of postoperative breast skin ischemia or necrosis is difficult to estimate, however, due to the lack of a standardized method to characterize the severity of ischemic tissue injury.

Mastectomy SKIN Score

A newly developed, simple scoring system assessing the severity of breast skin injury after mastectomy and IBR is now available: the Mastectomy SKIN Score (unpublished report). The Mastectomy SKIN Score was developed at Mayo Clinic by a group of breast surgeons and plastic surgeons as part of a quality improvement initiative seeking to reduce the morbidity of SSM or NSM with IBR. It is patterned after the established scoring system for burn injuries[24] (ie, a scoring system that takes into account both the depth and the extent of tissue injury). When using the Mastectomy SKIN Score, a score with 2 components is assigned to each operated breast (**Table 2**):

1. A letter score on a 4-point scale for depth of skin ischemic injury
   plus
2. A numeric score on a 4-point scale for the surface area of the deepest skin ischemic injury

The categories for depth of ischemic tissue injury include the extremes of no skin injury and full-thickness necrosis. Two intermediate categories for depth of injury are appointed: one for partial thickness necrosis that must demonstrate evidence of partial thickness necrosis by at least epidermal sloughing and a milder category of skin color change suggestive of ischemia (this could include cyanosis or erythema) in the absence of any findings of actual tissue necrosis. For assessing the size of the area involved, a parallel structure of 4 categories is selected:

1. None
2. 1%–10%
3. 11%–30%
4. Greater than 30%

In a retrospective review of consecutive patients who underwent SSM or NSM with IBR, postoperative photograph scores using the Mastectomy SKIN Score, including both the letter score (ie, depth of tissue ischemic injury) and the numeric score (ie, surface area involved) as well as their combinations, strongly correlated with reoperation outcomes. The combined letter and numeric score demonstrated a C statistic of 0.97 for SSM and 0.94 for NSM, for predicting need for additional

Table 2
Mastectomy SKIN Score. Each breast receives both a number and a letter score to characterize the severity of breast skin ischemic injury, based on 2 characteristics: (1) the greatest depth of tissue ischemic injury and (2) the surface area involved of the area of greatest depth. The breast mound and nipple-areolar complex are scored separately

Depth of Tissue Ischemic Injury		Surface Area Involved	
Score	Definition	Score	Definition
A	No evidence of skin ischemia or necrosis	1	None
B	Color change of skin suggesting impaired perfusion or ischemia (may be cyanosis or erythema)	2	Change involving 1%–10% of breast skin or 1%–10% of NAC
C	Partial thickness skin necrosis resulting in at least epidermal sloughing	3	Change involving 11%–30% of breast skin or 11%–30% of NAC or total nipple involvement[a]
D	Full-thickness skin necrosis[b]	4	Change involving > 30% of breast skin or > 30% of NAC

Abbreviation: NAC, nipple-areolar complex.

[a] Because the nipple itself is considered a key to the aesthetics of the breast, if there is skin necrosis involving the entire nipple, the surface area score of the NAC is automatically upgraded to a score of at least 3, even if the nipple represents less than 10% of the surface area of the NAC.

[b] Note: areas that are not definitely full thickness should be scored as partial thickness.

surgical intervention after breast skin ischemic injury (unpublished data). It is currently in the process of validation.

Donor Site Morbidity

In the setting of postmastectomy reconstruction, which procedure is chosen is often based on patient preferences for health outcomes and their risk profile. The most common type of autologous tissue breast reconstruction uses the abdominal donor to reconstruct the breast. Newer surgical techniques designed to decrease abdominal wall morbidity have led to an increasing number of women seeking microvascular transverse rectus abdominis myocutaneous (TRAM) or perforator flap reconstruction rather than traditional pedicled TRAM flap reconstruction. The relative benefit of these individual flaps remains, however, controversial.

Despite the lack of consensus in the literature regarding abdominal donor site morbidity in TRAM or related flap reconstruction patients, few argue that the donor site is often a source of patient anxiety and concern. Adequate levels of abdominal muscular strength are necessary to engage in daily activities, such as lifting, performing sports-related activity, and maintaining erect posture. That said, outcome data that evaluate potential donor site morbidity after autogenous tissue reconstruction should be incorporated into the informed consent process.

To date, the bulk of published data regarding abdominal donor site morbidity has used objective measures to evaluate isolated abdominal muscle function. The most common measurement tool used for this purpose is a dynamometer. Dynamometers are devices that measure force or power. Several classes of dynamometers are available for measuring isometric, isotonic, or isokinetic muscle strength. The isometric dynamometer requires an individual to push or pull maximally against the recording device without movement taking place. The isotonic dynamometer requires lifting as much weight as possible through a full range of motion. The isokinetic meter controls the speed of movement during maximal contraction while measuring the force applied.

Dynamometers are frequently used to assess neuromuscular function because they can, in theory, provide objective, detailed torque and velocity data—variables that can be used to calculate overall muscle strength. There is evidence, however, to suggest that the reliability of dynamometry depends on the muscle groups tested. For example, Agre and colleagues[25] found better reliability of isokinetic testing with upper limb muscles compared with lower limb muscles. To the best of the authors' knowledge, no group has evaluated the reliability of dynamometry in the breast reconstructive population. In a population of patients with chronic low back pain, reliability testing revealed highly significant learning effects for isometric trunk flexion and isokinetic abdominal measurements.[26] It has also been suggested that the use of a warm-up before and/or rest period between repeated measurements may influence the fatigability of a muscle and ultimately in the maximal strength recorded. It follows that using repeat measures to evaluate truncal function with these measurement tools may be problematic.

Perhaps given these issues, as well as the expense and complexity involved in using a dynamometer, other groups have simply used ability to do sit-ups as a surrogate measurement for formal strength testing.[27] More formal grading systems, such as the Kendall and the Lacote grading system, which similarly use clinical examination and manual muscle testing to evaluate function, have also been used in this setting (**Table 3**).[28] Hamdi and colleagues,[29] for example, evaluated 20 consecutive patients after 17 unilateral and 3 bilateral deep inferior epigastric perforator flap reconstructions for the purpose of measuring their abdominal wall function preoperatively and at 3 and 6 months postoperatively using a muscle grading system. Their results suggest that all patients had reached or even improved their preoperative level of upper and lower rectus muscle function 6 months after the operation. The external oblique muscles were the most affected by the procedure of flap harvesting, but only 2 patients were found to have a measurable impairment after 6 months.

Although the use of clinical examination and/or manual muscle testing is straightforward and easy to perform, neither of these approaches has undergone formal evaluation with respect to their ability to either produce consistent results or detect subtle differences between groups of well-performing subjects. Furthermore, there is concern that because the measurement is based on a provider's subjective observation, it may be imprecise and vulnerable to observer bias. In short, further research is needed to evaluate the psychometrics of the measurement tools used to measure abdominal strength in the breast reconstructive population and to determine which measures are associated with lower levels of measurement error.

Further consideration of an additional measurement challenge in this population is also warranted. At present, interpretation of the measurement of abdominal function in the population of women who undergo TRAM or related flap reconstructions poses a unique challenge in that extraordinary variability in both the amount of muscle that is injured and/or harvested during a pedicled TRAM, a free TRAM and a deep inferior epigastric perforator flap exists. From a measurement point of view, this allows for the introduction of significant bias into findings reported if populations of patients cannot be accurately classified and homogenous groups and cannot be created for the purposes of comparison.

PATIENT-REPORTED OUTCOMES

It is well known that objective measures do not always correlate with a patient's subjective experience or their assessment of the surgical outcome. Therefore, subjective data obtained through patient questionnaires or patient reported outcome instruments are critical.

To rigorously evaluate outcomes from a patient perspective, well-developed and validated patient

Table 3
Kendall grading of trunk muscle strength assessment

Trunk Curl (Lying, Feet Flat and Unsupported)	
Grade	Observed Ability
1	Unable to raise more than head off table
2	Arms extended toward knees, scapulae lifted from table
3	Arms straight, lumbar spine lifted from table
4	Arms crossed over chest, lumbar spine lifted from table
5	Hands behind neck, lumbar spine lifted from table

Leg Lowering (Angle Between Long Axis of Femur and Table, When Pelvis Begins to Tilt)	
Grade	Degrees
0	90—75
1	74—60
2	59—45
3	44—30
4	29—15
5	14—0

reported outcome (PROs) instruments must be used. PRO instruments designed to measure satisfaction and quality of life ask patients to report views, feelings, and experiences that are unavoidably personal phenomena. Ideally, a PRO instrument designed to evaluate breast surgery patients' perception of outcome should

1. Address breast surgery–specific issues and
2. Undergo full development and validation as outlined by the Scientific Advisory Committee of the Medical Outcomes Trust and Food and Drug Administration guidance

Historically, a lack of reliable, valid, breast surgery–specific questionnaires existed. Instead, researchers relied on either ad hoc questionnaires that were neither formally developed nor tested or on well-developed, validated questionnaires that were not specific to the breast surgery population. Although these later instruments often proved psychometrically sound, in most cases, they were not sensitive enough to capture all aspects of the outcome specific to a particular breast procedure.

Chen and colleagues[30] recently illustrated this point. A systematic review was performed to identify existing instruments that addressed some aspect of a patient's subjective experience with oncologic breast surgery (lumpectomy, mastectomy, or breast reconstruction). Ten PRO instruments were identified and evaluated. Their group concluded that both the European Organisation for Research and Treatment of Cancer QLQ-BR23 and the FACT-B are well-developed instruments that have been extensively tested among breast cancer patients. These commonly used and widely accepted PROs are disease specific rather than surgery specific, which decreases their ability to evaluate change brought about by surgery of the breast (ie, changes in nipple sensation, firmness around an implant, and donor site morbidity). Five additional measures (Polivy BIS, Breast Cancer Treatment Outcome Scale, Mastectomy Attitude Scale, and 2 Michigan Breast Reconstruction Outcome Study questionnaires) seem to address relevant breast surgery–related issues but fail to demonstrate evidence of a rigorous development process and/or formal psychometric evaluation. In contrast, the HBIS, BIBCQ, and BREAST-Q seem well-developed PRO measures that address breast surgery–specific issues. The investigators caution, however, that although the BIBCQ addresses issues relating to body image after mastectomy and lumpectomy, it is limited in its assessment of the impact of breast reconstruction.

Their team notes that the BREAST-Q is the only questionnaire that used new psychometric technology (ie, Rasch) in its development. This new methodology allowed for the creation of a PRO instrument that is valid for use both in performing population-based research and evaluating individual patients in real time. As such, it creates a measurement tool that is suitable for use in routine clinical care and may allow surgeons to be more effective in addressing the specific issues of a patient.

The BREAST-Q was designed with a modular, procedure-specific structure (reconstruction, reduction, and augmentation); each procedure-specific module has a preoperative and postoperative version and the same conceptual model. The scale structure of the BREAST-Q addresses both quality of life (psychosocial well-being, physical well-being, and sexual well-being) and patient satisfaction (satisfaction with breasts, satisfaction with outcome, and satisfaction with process of care). A Likert-type response format is used. Items in each scale are summed and transformed on a 0 to 100 scale, with higher values representing a more favorable outcome. Psychometric evaluation of individual scales has shown high levels of internal consistency and test-retest reliability. Hypothesis testing for the reconstruction module (known group differences with respect to patient age, implant type, autologous vs implant reconstruction, and radiation history) has confirmed construct validity of the scales (see the article by Cano and colleagues elsewhere in this issue).[31,32]

NATIONAL OUTCOME AUDITS IN BREAST SURGERY
National Surgical Quality Improvement Project

The NSQIP is a national, data-driven, risk-adjusted, outcomes-based surgical quality improvement program to assist health care organizations in building the foundation for benchmarking and comparing clinical outcomes within an institution and to other participating health care organizations. It originated in the Veterans Health Administration and has been operational since 1991.[33–36] In 2001, the American College of Surgeons received funding to implement the NSQIP pilot program in private sector hospitals, and the program was expanded in 2004 to additional private sector hospitals. To date, NSQIP is considered the best, most comprehensive, and accurate national surgical database that houses, measures, and reports surgical outcomes data. It captures morbidity variables for specific surgical procedures and calculates expected morbidity probabilities. It allows identification of outcome differences and opportunities for practice convergence with the ultimate goal of improving patient care and surgical outcomes while decreasing institutional health care costs. NSQIP collects data on 136 variables, inclusive of the preoperative risk factors and intraoperative and 30-day postoperative morbidity and mortality outcomes for patients undergoing major surgical procedures in both the inpatient and the outpatient settings. Because it applies for breast surgery performed by plastic surgeons, NSQIP targets the following procedures: tissue flaps, breast reductions, and breast reconstruction.

Studies based on NSQIP data

To date, only a small number of studies have queried the NSQIP database from a plastic surgery perspective. In 2012, Ogunleye and colleagues reported the 30-day postoperative morbidity of delayed breast reconstruction. From 2005 to 2008, a cohort of 645 patients was identified in the NSQIP database. Of these, 67.6% of patients underwent implant-based breast reconstruction (implant alone or tissue expander placement), 19.1% of patients underwent breast reconstruction with pedicled TRAM flap, 9% of patients underwent breast reconstruction with latissimus dorsi myocutaneous flap, and only 3.6% of patients underwent microsurgical breast reconstruction. Surgical site infection was the most commonly reported complication, with a 5.7% rate. The investigators reported that body mass index greater than 25 and prior radiation treatment within 90 days were the only two statistically significant risk factors for development of wound infection on multivariate analysis. This data analysis is not procedure specific but instead examines combined outcomes of delayed prosthetic and autologous breast reconstruction procedures. Another recent study by Lovely and colleagues reviewed an NSQIP dataset from 2006 to 2010 for venous thromboembolic events (in patients undergoing breast surgery). For all NSQIP sites, a higher incidence of venous thromboembolic events was observed in patients undergoing mastectomy with IBR (0.3%) compared with patients undergoing mastectomy without reconstruction (0.2%), although this difference was not statistically significant ($P = .07$). These results are used to guide institutional venous thromboprophylaxis guidelines in an effort to reduce morbidity.

Limitations to NSQIP

The NSQIP dataset is not without drawbacks. One of the limitations of NSQIP is that it collects a sample size of approximately 20% of all surgical cases.

More specifically, each participating hospital center provides data on the first 20 consecutive surgical procedures in an 8-day cycle. Although this sample size is large enough to identify opportunities for improvement, it is not complete. Achieving 100% data collection, however, would require significantly more resources and be cost prohibitive. Another limitation of the NSQIP database is that due to its generic nature, it does not capture specialty-specific or procedure-specific variables.

SUMMARY

Current health care reforms in the United States require increasing transparency and accountability for health care outcomes. Knowledge about the strengths and weaknesses of available outcomes-based measures is essential to plastic surgeons, to ensure proper instrument selection and interpretation.

REFERENCES

1. Leonardi MC, Garusi C, Santoro L, et al. Impact of medical discipline and observer gender on cosmetic outcome evaluation in breast reconstruction using transverse rectus abdominis myocutaneous (TRAM) flap and radiotherapy. J Plast Reconstr Aesthet Surg 2010;63(12):2091–7.
2. Parliament MB, Danjoux CE, Clayton T. Is cancer treatment toxicity accurately reported? Int J Radiat Oncol Biol Phys 1985;11(3):603–8.
3. Basch E, Artz D, Dulko D, et al. Patient online self-reporting of toxicity symptoms during chemotherapy. J Clin Oncol 2005;23(15):3552–61.
4. Neben-Wittich MA, Atherton PJ, Schwartz DJ, et al. Comparison of provider-assessed and patient-reported outcome measures of acute skin toxicity during a Phase III trial of mometasone cream versus placebo during breast radiotherapy: the North Central Cancer Treatment Group (N06C4). Int J Radiat Oncol Biol Phys 2011;81(2):397–402.
5. Rose MA, Olivotto I, Cady B, et al. Conservative surgery and radiation therapy for early breast cancer. Long-term cosmetic results. Arch Surg 1989;124(2):153–7.
6. Kijima Y, Yoshinaka H, Funasako Y, et al. Immediate breast reconstruction using autologous free dermal fat grafts provides better cosmetic results for patients with upper inner cancerous lesions. Surg Today 2011;41(4):477–89.
7. Ueda S, Tamaki Y, Yano K, et al. Cosmetic outcome and patient satisfaction after skin-sparing mastectomy for breast cancer with immediate reconstruction of the breast. Surgery 2008;143(3):414–25.
8. Lowery JC, Wilkins EG, Kuzon WM, et al. Evaluations of aesthetic results in breast reconstruction: an

analysis of reliability. Ann Plast Surg 1996;36(6): 601–6 [discussion: 607].

9. Viera AJ, Garrett JM. Understanding interobserver agreement: the kappa statistic. Fam Med 2005; 37(5):360–3.

10. Landis JR, Koch GG. The measurement of observer agreement for categorical data. Biometrics 1977; 33(1):159–74.

11. Carlson GW, Page AL, Peters K, et al. Effects of radiation therapy on pedicled transverse rectus abdominis myocutaneous flap breast reconstruction. Ann Plast Surg 2008;60(5):568–72.

12. Spear SL, Baker JL Jr. Classification of capsular contracture after prosthetic breast reconstruction. Plast Reconstr Surg 1995;96(5):1119–23.

13. Zahavi A, Sklair ML, Ad-El DD. Capsular contracture of the breast: working towards a better classification using clinical and radiologic assessment. Ann Plast Surg 2006;57(3):248–51.

14. Siggelkow W, Faridi A, Spiritus K, et al. Histological analysis of silicone breast implant capsules and correlation with capsular contracture. Biomaterials 2003;24(6):1101–9.

15. Alfano C, Mazzocchi M, Scuderi N. Mammary compliance: an objective measurement of capsular contracture. Aesthetic Plast Surg 2004;28(2):75–9.

16. Gylbert L, Berggren A. Constant compression caliper for objective measurement of breast capsular contracture. Scand J Plast Reconstr Surg Hand Surg 1989; 23(2):137–42.

17. Gylbert LO. Applanation tonometry for the evaluation of breast compressibility. Scand J Plast Reconstr Surg Hand Surg 1989;23(3):223–9.

18. Garwood ER, Moore D, Ewing C, et al. Total skin-sparing mastectomy: complications and local recurrence rates in 2 cohorts of patients. Ann Surg 2009; 249(1):26–32.

19. Peled AW, Foster RD, Stover AC, et al. Outcomes after total skin-sparing mastectomy and immediate reconstruction in 657 breasts. Ann Surg Oncol 2012;19(11):3402–9.

20. Wijayanayagam A, Kumar AS, Foster RD, et al. Optimizing the total skin-sparing mastectomy. Arch Surg 2008;143(1):38–45.

21. Brooke S, Mesa J, Uluer M, et al. Complications in tissue expander breast reconstruction: a comparison of AlloDerm, DermaMatrix, and FlexHD acellular inferior pole dermal slings. Ann Plast Surg 2012; 69(4):347–9.

22. Moyer HR, Ghazi B, Daniel JR, et al. Nipple-sparing mastectomy: technical aspects and aesthetic outcomes. Ann Plast Surg 2012;68(5):446–50.

23. Moyer HR, Losken A. Predicting mastectomy skin flap necrosis with indocyanine green angiography:

the gray area defined. Plast Reconstr Surg 2012; 129(5):1043–8.

24. American Burn Association White Paper. Surgical management of the burn wound and use of skin substitutes. 2009. Available at: http://www.ameri-burn.org. Accessed January 20, 2012.

25. Agre JC, Magness JL, Hull SZ, et al. Strength testing with a portable dynamometer: reliability for upper and lower extremities. Arch Phys Med Rehabil 1987;68(7):454–8.

26. Hutten MM, Hermens HJ. Reliability of lumbar dynamometry measurements in patients with chronic low back pain with test-retest measurements on different days. Eur Spine J 1997;6(1):54–62.

27. Kroll SS, Schusterman MA, Reece GP, et al. Abdominal wall strength, bulging, and hernia after TRAM flap breast reconstruction. Plast Reconstr Surg 1995;96:616–9.

28. Atisha D, Alderman AK. A systematic review of abdominal wall function following abdominal flaps for postmastectomy breast reconstruction [review]. Ann Plast Surg 2009;63(2):222–30.

29. Hamdi M, Weiler-Moithoff EM, Webster MH. Deep inferior epigastric perforator flap in breast reconstruction: experience with the first 50 flaps. Plast Reconstr Surg 1999;103:86–95.

30. Chen CM, Cano SJ, Klassen AF, et al. Measuring quality of life in oncologic breast surgery: a systematic review of patient-reported outcome measures. Breast J 2010;16(6):587–97.

31. Pusic AL, Klassen AF, Scott AM, et al. Development of a new patient-reported outcome measure for breast surgery: the BREAST-Q. Plast Reconstr Surg 2009;124(2):345–53.

32. Cano SJ, Klassen AF, Scott AM, et al. The BREAST-Q: further validation in independent clinical samples. Plast Reconstr Surg 2012;129(2):293–302.

33. Khuri SF, Daley J, Henderson W, et al. The National Veterans Administration Surgical Risk Study: risk adjustment for the comparative assessment of the quality of surgical care. J Am Coll Surg 1995; 180(5):519–31.

34. American College of Surgeons. National surgical quality improvement program. 2008. Available at: http://site.acsnsqip.org/. Accessed August 8, 2012.

35. Ogunleye AA, de Blacam C, Curtis MS, et al. An analysis of delayed breast reconstruction outcomes as recorded in the American College of Surgeons National Surgical Quality Improvement Program. J Plast Reconstr Aesthet Surg 2012;65(3):289–94.

36. Lovely JK, Nehring SA, Boughey JC, et al. Balancing venous thromboembolism and hematoma after breast surgery. Ann Surg Oncol 2012;19(10): 3230–5.

Measuring Health-related Quality of Life Outcomes in Head and Neck Reconstruction

Claudia R. Albornoz, MD, MSc[a],
Andrea L. Pusic, MD, MHS, FRCSC[a], Patrick Reavey, MD[a],
Amie M. Scott, MPH[a], Anne F. Klassen, DPhil[b],
Stefan J. Cano, PhD[c], Peter G. Cordeiro, MD[a],
Evan Matros, MD, MMSc[a],*

KEYWORDS

- Quality of life[mesh] • Outcome assessment (health care)[mesh] • Head and neck neoplasms[mesh]
- Patient satisfaction[mesh] • Reconstructive surgical procedures [mesh] • Qualitative research[mesh]
- Patient-reported outcomes • Reconstruction

KEY POINTS

- Health-related quality of life is an important outcome following head and neck (H&N) reconstruction.
- Existing PRO instruments specific for H&N reconstruction have both methodological and content deficiencies.
- Qualitative interviews in 26 patients with H&N cancer showed content deficiencies in function following midface surgery (eg, oral competence, rhinorrhea, facial sensation, smile, vision, and eye discharge) and impact of altered facial appearance.
- The information obtained from the current study serves as the framework for item generation of a new pro instrument for patients with H&N cancers: the FACE-Q oncology.

PROBLEM OVERVIEW

It is estimated that there will be 42,870 new cases of head and neck (H&N) cancer in the United States in 2012.[1] Diagnosis and treatment can be stressful for patients and families, affecting physical, emotional, and psychological well-being.[2,3] Although quantitative end points such as mortality and recurrence time are measures of treatment success, there are other relevant aspects to consider.[4] Health-related quality of life (HR-QOL) is a multidimensional concept that, in oral cancer, includes aspects such as function, emotions, socialization, symptoms, expectations, and satisfaction.[4,5] HR-

QOL is increasingly recognized as an important outcome by the Agency for Healthcare Research and Quality and should be an integral component of plastic surgery outcomes.[6,7]

Patient-reported outcomes (PRO) instruments are questionnaires designed to gather information from patients about their physical, mental, and social well-being.[8] Although many PRO instruments for H&N reconstruction are currently in use, a systematic review identified both methodological and content deficiencies.[9] First, many of the H&N PRO instruments lacked patient input during generation. Outcomes considered to be important by clinicians

Disclosure: Part of this work was funded by a grant from the Plastic Surgery Foundation to Dr Pusic.
[a] Plastic and Reconstructive Surgical Service, Memorial Sloan-Kettering Cancer Center, 1275 York Avenue, MRI 1007, New York, NY 10065, USA; [b] Faculty of Health Sciences, McMaster University, 1280 Main street West, Hamilton L854K1, Canada; [c] Peninsula College of Medicine and Dentistry, Tamar Science Park, Davy Road. Room N13, ITTC Building 1, Plymouth PL6 8BX, UK
* Corresponding author. Moriemal Sloan-Kettering Cancer Center, 1275 York Avenue, MRI 1036, New York, NY 10065.
E-mail address: matrose@mskcc.org

may be incongruous with those of patients.[10,11] Second, existing PRO instruments measure some functional aspects following H&N surgery (eg, speech quality following glossectomy), but fail to measure psychosocial aspects (eg, social isolation related to unintelligible speech).[12,13] Third, even though facial disfigurement is one of the most stressful aspects of surgical resection, assessment of its impact is lacking.[9,14,15] Based on these findings, a more comprehensive PRO instrument is needed.

This article identifies, from the patient perspective, health and appearance concerns following H&N reconstruction. This qualitative approach serves as the foundation for development of a new PRO instrument.

METHODOLOGY
Participants

Following approval from the Memorial Sloan-Kettering Cancer Center Institutional Review Board, a qualitative study was performed. Eligible subjects were identified from the institutional database of patients with H&N cancer. Participants were required to have had reconstruction for cancer of the H&N region (**Table 1**). Purposive sampling was used to select the study population, including patients with different pathologic subtypes and disease locations, to ensure a heterogeneous H&N cancer population.

Patients were recruited by their plastic or oncologic surgeon by mail or during clinic appointments. Interested patients received documents describing the study and discussed participation with the research team. Patients who agreed to participate completed consent forms before interviews. They were free to withdraw from the study at any time. A total of 26 patients were interviewed.

Interviews

In-depth semistructured interviews that lasted approximately 1 hour were conducted by experienced qualitative researchers (AS, PR) at the hospital. An interview guide was designed based on the H&N cancer literature, content included in currently available H&N PRO instruments, and suggestions from an expert panel of plastic surgeons (**Box 1**). Interviews were recorded digitally and transcribed verbatim without patient identifiers.

Data Analysis

Data collection and analysis took place concurrently, which allowed modifications of the interview guide to gather data to refine emerging codes. Sample size was determined by saturation (when no new emergent themes appeared). Transcripts were coded line by line to examine, compare, and develop conceptual categories. Categories were developed inductively using the constant comparison method. Each item was compared with the rest of the data to create analytical categories. They were grouped to identify key themes. Coding was discussed during regular meetings with the research team.

EVIDENCE

Characteristics of the 26 interviewees are shown in **Table 2**. Most patients had a midface reconstruction (41%), followed by the lower face (27%) and upper face (22%).

Analysis identified several important concerns for patients with H&N cancers, which were categorized into the following main themes (**Fig. 1**):

- Altered facial function and psychosocial impact
- Altered facial appearance and psychosocial impact
- Mediators

Altered Facial Function and Psychosocial Impact

This category describes functional changes with associated sequelae after H&N surgery. Patients reported functional concerns in the following areas: speech, salivation, eating, facial sensation,

---

Table 1
Patient inclusion and exclusion criteria

Inclusion Criteria	Exclusion Criteria
Age 18–80 y old	Inability to speak or participate in interview
Surgical reconstruction following resection of H&N cancer: free, local, and regional flaps	Cognitive impairment or active psychiatric illness that would prevent patient from participating in interview
Follow-up from 6 wk to 7 y following latest resection	Primary closure of surgical defect
Resection/reconstruction resulting in alteration in facial appearance	

Box 1
Interview guide

Early/background questions: experience after diagnosis, therapies received

Process of care/preparedness questions: preparation for surgery, information about reconstruction from physicians, seeking of additional information, satisfaction with information, satisfaction with care

Facial function: changes in expressions or function

Facial appearance: changes in facial appearance, feelings about appearance, satisfaction with facial appearance

Social functioning/situations: work, public, social activities, relationships

Psychological functioning: feelings about themselves, mood, self-confidence, body image

Expectations: fulfillment of expectations, willingness to have additional procedures

Coping: strategies

Other aspects not covered

Table 2
Clinical and demographic characteristics of the interviewed patients

Characteristics	n (%)
Age (years)	
30–45	7 (27)
46–60	5 (19)
>60	14 (54)
Gender	
Female	14 (54)
Male	12 (46)
Caucasian	15 (58)
Other	11 (42)
Histology	
Sarcoma	4 (15)
Melanoma	5 (19)
Squamous cell carcinoma (oral cavity)	9 (35)
Squamous cell carcinoma (skin)	4 (15)
Basal cell carcinoma	3 (12)
Other	1 (4)
Oncologic surgery	
Mandibulectomy	5 (19)
Maxillectomy	8 (31)
Midface skin and/or soft tissue resection	11 (42)
Neck soft tissue resection	2 (8)
Main Reconstructive Surgery	
Microsurgical Flaps	15 (58)
Fibula flap	5
Rectus abdominis flap	5
Parascapular flap	2
Radial forearm flap	2
Anterolateral thigh flap	1
Pedicled or Local Flaps	11 (42)
Temporalis muscle flap	3
Forehead flap	2
Adjacent tissue transfer (eg, cheek flap)	3
Full-thickness skin graft	3
Follow-up (y)	
Mean (range)	1.48 (0.3–5.0)

oral competence, runny nose, tearing, vision, and smiling (**Fig. 2**). Most impairment in facial function had an associated psychosocial impact, which contributed to social anxiety and difficulty interacting with people.

Speech

Speech impairment was related to decreased mouth opening, decreased salivation, tongue immobility, and mouth stiffness. Speech changes were common in the period immediately following surgery, but improved over time for many patients. Speech difficulties ranged from minor pronunciation problems to an ability to communicate only with family members. Patients complained that their mouths did not move or open sufficiently to pronounce certain sounds or words. Difficulties with speech comprehension, both in person and on the telephone, were commonly described.

"Certain letters would get stuck because that (mouth) opening wasn't over far enough."
"My speech doesn't sound right."

Changes in speech altered self-confidence. Patients described that they were more self-conscious, nervous, frustrated, and/or embarrassed when they could not be understood. In the extreme form, patients avoided speaking, which contributed to degrees of social isolation.

"...And that (speech) can get a little embarrassing at times. I can be talking to someone and all of a sudden realize, wow, my speech doesn't sound right."

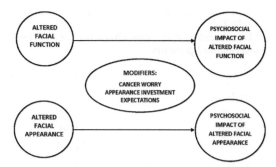

Fig. 1. Conceptual model of health-related quality of life after H&N cancer reconstruction.

Salivation

Lack of saliva was a problem for patients with radiotherapy history. Dry mouth was reported to cause difficulty with both speech and eating. Some patients required liquids to eat.

Eating

Eating problems were related to sensory changes of the tongue/lips/mucosa, lack of saliva, oral incompetence, abnormal mouth opening, lack of teeth, and swallowing difficulty. Specific food items were challenging to eat (eg, hamburger, vegetables). Some patients could only eat food cut into small pieces or pureed. Drinking from a cup was also reported to be difficult. Eating and drinking required significant effort and took an extended amount of time compared with before surgery. Certain foods or drinks often lacked taste because of radiotherapy side effects.

"It's hard for me to bite into things. It's hard for me to manage food because I also have a loss of feeling on my tongue."

"They took a lot of teeth out, so I have to cut my food very small. I can't eat things I like to eat."

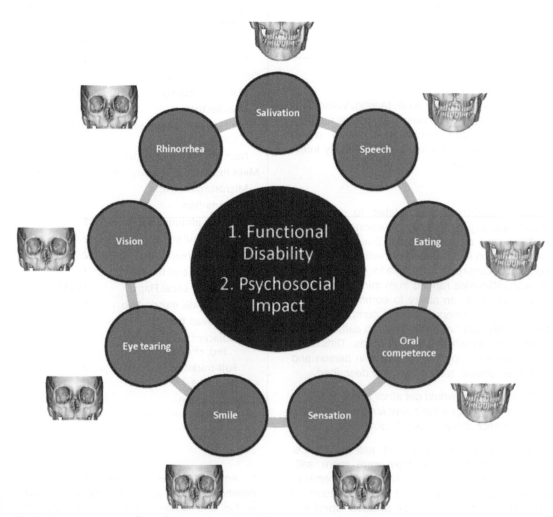

Fig. 2. Functional areas affected in patients after H&N cancer reconstruction.

Eating and/or drinking in public were stressful for many patients. The inability to eat normally was a source of embarrassment for many participants, preventing them from engaging in social activities that included food or drink. Eating was no longer an enjoyable social activity.

"I can't always tell where food is in my mouth because I can't feel it. I can't tell if it's spilling out of my mouth…so I'm very conscious during those situations."

"We used to go out to eat. Right now I'm just not comfortable going to a restaurant, really…because you don't know how the food's going to be, how I am going to be able to handle it."

Facial sensation
Altered facial sensation or reconstructive flap numbness made it challenging for participants to know whether food, nasal secretions, or tears were on their face.

"I can have food on my lips or chin and I don't even know. I don't know that I need to wipe with a napkin or I can't feel that it was dribbling out of my mouth. Normal things that other people who can feel don't even think about."

Numbness was a significant source of social anxiety. Participants were concerned about how other people interpreted physical signs such as tears on their face. Sometimes participants avoided social interaction.

"The very first time it (drooling) happened was in the context of my family and it was so humiliating….It was so embarrassing that I felt like, you know, I'm sitting there like some demented elderly person, drooling, spittle hanging out of my mouth…and I'm clueless…"

Oral competence
Oral incompetence was caused by mechanical and neurologic changes following surgery, including numbness, scars, bulky flaps, and muscular paralysis. Patients complained of drooling at rest and difficulty processing food during meals.

"You know, I think my lip is a major thing for eating. I still use a straw a lot of times…Because it's (my lip) pulled over."

Rhinorrhea
Rhinorrhea was reported, commonly in association with numbness. Participants could not feel nasal secretions on their faces so they were constantly wiping their noses.

"And it's an extreme embarrassment to me if I were out socially and suddenly this discharge is running out my nose and I'm sitting here elegantly talking to somebody."

Eye discharge
Eye discharge was related to blocked or absent tear ducts following surgery or radiotherapy. It was especially problematic for women because they could not wear makeup. Tearing was also embarrassing because people misinterpreted it as crying or illness.

"There's a discharge from my eye. …say you're sitting next to somebody in a theater or something so close and they see, you know, this little goo coming out of your eye, they may think you're ill or something."

Vision
Visual changes, such as double vision and absent depth perception, were related to periorbital surgery following maxillectomy reconstruction. Participants complained of blurred vision, that their eyes got tired easily, or that they had difficulty walking down stairs, reading, and driving. Vision problems made people feel disabled because of their dependency on other persons to assist with activities like driving and cooking.

Smile
Participants complained their smile appeared like a grimace, crooked, odd, or lopsided and no longer effectively conveyed the intended emotion. Furthermore, during animation, an abnormal smile drew attention to postsurgical changes by highlighting asymmetries. Participants became self-conscious, insecure, or embarrassed, and reported that they smiled less than before surgery.

Altered Facial Appearance and Psychosocial Impact

In general, participants were not as concerned with minute aesthetic aspects of facial appearance following reconstruction as they were with their overall facial appearance. Facial asymmetry was a key issue because it accentuated differences between the unaffected side and postsurgical abnormalities.

"My jaw was crooked."
"My face went to one side"
"I should say the less symmetry you have because of an operation, the more, the heavier

the load of anxiety and so forth. Because it's not a scar...it's being disfigured. Something's out of place. That's noticed much more than a discoloration."

To a lesser extent, participants were bothered by alterations in facial contour, color, and scarring, because it drew attention to the surgical site. Attempts were made to camouflage changes with makeup, scarves, glasses, and hats. In some instance, these differences improved over time.

"When it doesn't flare red, I can camouflage it. But when it flares red, I really can't camouflage it."
"There's a thickness and puffiness in my flap."
"It was all bumpy and lumpy."
"I have a sunken part on my face."

When present, functional impairments were a priority relative to changes in appearance. In the absence of functional problems, patients focused on changes in the way they looked.

"I don't think that being disfigured...would really bother me as long as I was able to communicate and eat and just do my work..."
"I've never had a problem with adjusting to my appearance. I've never even thought about it...It's been more the fact that I can't taste and smell things."

Regardless of the nature of the alteration in facial appearance (color difference, contour abnormality, or scarring), the common psychosocial impact of reconstructive surgery was decreased self-confidence and increased social anxiety. These findings were observed in participants with major or minor defects. Participants worried about other people's reactions to their altered facial appearance. They were stressed about how to resume participation in activities that require face-to-face interaction. They expressed feeling self-conscious, anxious, insecure, and embarrassed about their appearance. The impact of social anxiety ranged from patients who were aware of changes in physical appearance but continued to engage socially to those who avoided family and friends.

"I worry that I look a little silly...I feel silly smiling because maybe I look a little goofy or a little odd."
"I'm always conscious that someone's looking at my eye. And even if you're not, I'm conscious...I'm thinking people are saying what's the matter with her eye? It's

crooked...a lot of that may be in my own head, but it bothers me."

Participants reported low self-esteem following surgery because they felt different. The initial impression of scar size was shocking, but confidence increased as postsurgical changes improved. Over time, many patients adapted to the change and eventually were able to accept their altered appearance.

"It didn't look pretty at first. I was scared of myself...but when it started healing, it started looking much better."
"I would not be regarded as attractive...on the same level of attractiveness (as before)...there is a diminishment of self-confidence about my appearance...I don't feel as attractive."

Mediators

Mediators are factors that either ameliorate or exacerbate the impact of functional and/or appearance alterations following H&N reconstructive surgery. Three mediators were frequently identified during the interviews: cancer worry, appearance investment, and expectations.

Cancer worry

Fear of cancer affected the relative value placed on facial function and appearance. Immediately before surgery, participants were so afraid of cancer that they wanted it removed regardless of the surgical sequelae. As the disease-free interval lengthened, subjects had increased awareness of facial function and appearance.

"I was given information, but I didn't hear it. ...everything was clouded by fear."
"The surgeons kept saying this is going to affect your appearance. Your skin colors may not match up, but when you put it in perspective, that was very trivial compared with the cancer continuing to grow."

Appearance investment

Participants who cared greatly about their appearance before surgery were more likely to be negatively affected by their altered physical appearance.

"My appearance has been a part of how I've earned my living and how I've identified myself...it is a part of who I am, how I look like is very important to my career."

Expectations

Expectations correlate inversely to the level of satisfaction with postoperative appearance and

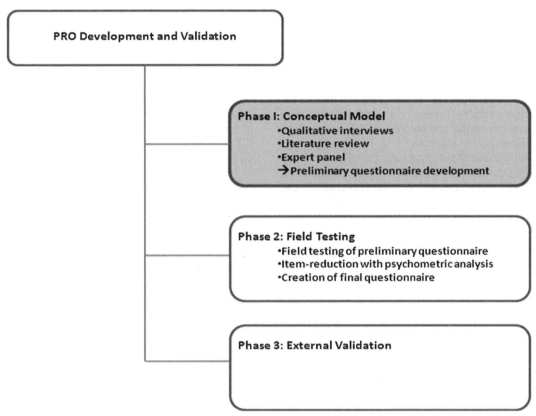

Fig. 3. Phases of PRO development.

function. Participants with high expectations were more likely to be dissatisfied because of a mismatch between their preconceived outcome and what can be achieved with reconstruction.

> "I was not prepared for the scars. I wasn't. I just assumed it would be a small scar."
> "If I knew exactly what it looked like, I probably never would have done it, to be honest with you."

SUMMARY

The strength of qualitative methodology is its ability to gather information about relevant issues from people affected by the sequelae of disease. This information provides the foundation for any instrument that attempts to evaluate patient HR-QOL. The current study confirms the findings of a previous systematic review: existing PRO instruments incompletely evaluate many meaningful problems for patients with H&N cancers.[9]

Following H&N cancer ablation and reconstruction, patients described disabilities in 9 facial functions. Several symptoms related to midface surgery, such as facial sensation, oral competence, rhinorrhea, eye tearing, vision, and smile, are missing from existing PRO instruments. This omission may reflect that current PRO H&N instruments were developed with input from patients undergoing lower face (mandible and tongue) or neck (pharynx and larynx) surgery.[16–24] The inclusion of midface symptoms would provide a more comprehensive measure of HR-QOL for patients who have H&N surgery. Each specific functional disability was also associated with degrees of psychosocial impairment ranging from self-awareness to social isolation. In general, the extent of functional disability correlated with the degree of psychosocial distress.

Facial appearance alterations were an important concern for patients following H&N reconstruction. Contrary to our expectations, participants were not overly concerned with scars, flap color, or contour, but were concerned with big-picture changes in facial appearance. Asymmetry was the most important concern, because it accentuated differences between the affected and normal sides of their faces. Changes in facial appearance created substantial psychosocial distress ranging from lack of self-confidence to avoidance of family and friends. Several reports suggest that facial appearance is a major concern in long-term oral cancer survivors, leading to changes in self-esteem, problems with partners, sexuality, and social isolation, but existing PRO instruments do not comprehensively assess its impact.[3,9,15,16,20,25–29] In addition, with increasing use of facial allotransplantation for correction of severe facial deformities, outcomes of these procedures need to be scientifically measured. Content from the current and additional interviews will serve as the framework for PRO instruments development in this area.

An additional set of factors, termed mediators, were identified that ameliorated or exacerbated the effect of changes in function and appearance. For example, patients were less concerned about function and appearance early in their treatment course because of preoccupation with survival. The concept of cancer worry identified is also included in other PRO instruments, including the Functional Assessment of Cancer Therapy - Head and Neck and the Head and Neck Cancer Inventory.[15,17] Cancer worry may exemplify response shift whereby health changes cause a shift of internal standards, values, and conceptualization. Response shift is important because it can distort the interpretation of changes in HR-QOL scores over time. Although none of the existing H&N PRO instruments incorporate appearance investment or expectations, inclusion of these concepts may help to understand variation in outcomes within patient groups.

According to the guidelines of the Scientific Advisory Committee of the Medical Outcomes Trust, the 3-stage development process for PRO instruments should include development of a conceptual model with question generation (stage I), field testing of the questionnaire (stage II), and psychometric analysis (stage III) (**Fig. 3**).[30] Qualitative research is the primary source of information for stage I. The information obtained from the current study serves as the framework for item generation of a new PRO instrument for patients with H&N cancers: the reconstructive module for the FACE-Q.[15] In an era of patient-centered treatments, accurate measurement of the extent and impact of symptoms following H&N reconstructive surgery is crucial to adjust treatment and rehabilitation to patient needs.[5,11] With increasing focus on evidence-based medicine and cost-effectiveness, PRO instruments are an important data source to justify many of the interventions performed by plastic and reconstructive surgeons.

REFERENCES

1. Siegel R, Naishadham D, Jemal A. Cancer statistics, 2012. CA Cancer J Clin 2012;62:10–29.

2. Roing M, Hirsch JM, Holmstrom I. Living in a state of suspension–a phenomenological approach to the spouse's experience of oral cancer. Scand J Caring Sci 2008;22:40–7.

3. Moore R, Chamberlain R, Khuri F. A qualitative study of head and neck cancer. Support Care Cancer 2004;12:338–46.

4. Chandu A, Smith AC, Rogers SN. Health-related quality of life in oral cancer: a review. J Oral Maxillofac Surg 2006;64:495–502.

5. Tschiesner U, Linseisen E, Coenen M, et al. Evaluating sequelae after head and neck cancer from the patient perspective with the help of the International Classification of Functioning, Disability and Health. Eur Arch Otorhinolaryngol 2009;266:425–36.

6. AHRQ-National Quality Measures Clearinghouse. Quality measures: patient-reported outcomes for quality improvement of clinical practice. 2012. Available at: http://qualitymeasures.ahrq.gov/expert/printView.aspx?id=36851. Accessed May 1, 2012.

7. Davis Sears E, Chung KC. A guide to interpreting a study of patient-reported outcomes. Plast Reconstr Surg 2012;129:1200–7.

8. US Food and Drug Administration. Patient-reported outcome measures: use in medical product development to support labeling claims. 2009. Available at: http://www.ispor.org/workpaper/FDA%20PRO%20Guidance.pdf. Accessed January 15, 2012.

9. Pusic A, Liu JC, Chen CM, et al. A systematic review of patient-reported outcome measures in head and neck cancer surgery. Otolaryngol Head Neck Surg 2007;136:525–35.

10. Turpin M, Dallos R, Owen R, et al. The meaning and impact of head and neck cancer: an interpretative phenomenological and repertory grid analysis. J Constr Psychol 2009;22:24–54.

11. Lee EW, Twinn S, Moore AP, et al. Clinical encounter experiences of patients with nasopharyngeal carcinoma. Integr Cancer Ther 2008;7:24–32.

12. Hartl DM, Dauchy S, Escande C, et al. Quality of life after free-flap tongue reconstruction. J Laryngol Otol 2009;123:550–4.

13. Bozec A, Poissonnet G, Chamorey E, et al. Free-flap head and neck reconstruction and quality of life: a 2-year prospective study. Laryngoscope 2008;118:874–80.

14. Katz MR, Irish JC, Devins GM, et al. Reliability and validity of an observer-rated disfigurement scale for head and neck cancer patients. Head Neck 2000;22:132–41.

15. Katre C, Johnson IA, Humphris GM, et al. Assessment of problems with appearance, following surgery for oral and oro-pharyngeal cancer using the University of Washington Appearance Domain and the Derriford Appearance Scale. Oral Oncol 2008;44:927–34.

16. Bjordal K, Ahlner-Elmqvist M, Tollesson E, et al. Development of a European Organization for Research and

Treatment of Cancer (EORTC) questionnaire module to be used in quality of life assessments in head and neck cancer patients. EORTC Quality of Life Study Group. Acta Oncol 1994;33:879–85.

17. Cella DF, Tulsky DS, Gray G, et al. The functional assessment of cancer therapy scale: development and validation of the general measure. J Clin Oncol 1993;11:570–9.

18. Terrell JE, Nanavati KA, Esclamado RM, et al. Head and neck cancer-specific quality of life: instrument validation. Arch Otolaryngol Head Neck Surg 1997; 123:1125–32.

19. Funk GF, Karnell LH, Christensen AJ, et al. Comprehensive head and neck oncology health status assessment. Head Neck 2003;25:561–75.

20. Rogers SN, Lowe D, Brown JS, et al. The University of Washington head and neck cancer measure as a predictor of outcome following primary surgery for oral cancer. Head Neck 1999;21:394–401.

21. Taylor RJ, Chepeha JC, Teknos TN, et al. Development and validation of the neck dissection impairment index: a quality of life measure. Arch Otolaryngol Head Neck Surg 2002;128:44–9.

22. Morton RP, Witterick IJ. Rationale and development of a quality-of-life instrument for head-and-neck cancer patients. Am J Otolaryngol 1995;16:284–93.

23. Gliklich RE, Goldsmith TA, Funk GF. Are head and neck specific quality of life measures necessary? Head Neck 1997;19:474–80.

24. List MA, Ritter-Sterr CA, Baker TM, et al. Longitudinal assessment of quality of life in laryngeal cancer patients. Head Neck 1996;18:1–10.

25. de Boer MF, Pruyn JF, van den Borne B, et al. Rehabilitation outcomes of long-term survivors treated for head and neck cancer. Head Neck 1995;17:503–15.

26. Semple C, McCance T. Experience of parents with head and neck cancer who are caring for young children. J Adv Nurs 2010;66:1280–90.

27. Larsson M, Hedelin B, Athlin E. A supportive nursing care clinic: conceptions of patients with head and neck cancer. Eur J Oncol Nurs 2007;11:49–59.

28. Strauss RP. Psychosocial responses to oral and maxillofacial surgery for head and neck cancer. J Oral Maxillofac Surg 1989;47:343–8.

29. Gamba A, Romano M, Grosso IM, et al. Psychosocial adjustment of patients surgically treated for head and neck cancer. Head Neck 1992;14: 218–23.

30. Scientific Advisory Committee of the Medical Outcomes, Trust. Assessing health status and quality-of-life instruments: attributes and review criteria. Qual Life Res 2002;11:193–205.

Future of Outcomes Research in Plastic Surgery

Toni Zhong, MD, MHS, FRCSC[a],*,
Andrea L. Pusic, MD, MPH, FRCSC[b]

KEYWORDS

- Outcomes research • Future directions • Study designs • PROs • Health services research

KEY POINTS

- Outcomes research, traditionally conducted on its own, has become integrated into clinical research, using clinical trial and observational study designs.
- Outcomes such as health-related quality of life and patient satisfaction can be studied as primary end points in clinical trials. However, well-designed randomized controlled trials (RCT) in plastic surgery are still limited because of the challenges of designing a surgical RCT.
- New methods in observational studies, such as propensity scores, the development of outcome measures such as valid and specific patient-reported outcome instruments, as well as the use of qualitative study designs, are advancing outcomes research.
- Health services research, which focuses on evaluation, is becoming increasing important to understand the associations between the need, supply, cost, and outcomes of care.

OVERVIEW

The assessment of outcomes has taken on new importance in many areas of plastic and reconstructive surgery in the last decade, and this point has been discussed in previous articles. Several driving factors such as the public's demand for more accountability, growing cost of health care, and emphasis on the value as well as impact of health services have culminated in an increased need for outcomes research. To address these broad issues, outcomes research differs from other medical research in that it is more inclusive of what is considered an intervention. Although most medical research examines the effects of a medication or surgical intervention, outcome research may examine the effects of counseling or the way care is delivered (process of care). As a result, outcome research is generally undertaken to address 1 of the following issues: (1) to help health care consumers make market decisions; (2) to assess the quality of medical care; or (3) to improve the knowledge base of medicine.[1]

The most striking shift in outcomes research has been its incorporation into mainstream clinical research, including its incorporation into clinical trials and observational studies.[2] In the past, the key features that distinguished clinical research from outcomes research was the emphasis on efficacy (effect of an intervention measured under the controlled circumstance of a clinical trial) as opposed to effectiveness (effect in the real world). However, with the infiltration of outcomes research into the mainstream clinical research,

Funding sources: Dr Zhong, Conquer Cancer Foundation and ASCO, CBCF, ASRM. Dr Pusic, none.
Conflict of interest: Dr Zhong, Nil. Dr Pusic is codeveloper of the BREAST-Q.
[a] Division of Plastic and Reconstructive Surgery, Department of Surgery and Surgical Oncology, University of Toronto, Toronto, Ontario, Canada; [b] Plastic and Reconstructive Surgical Service, Memorial Sloan-Kettering Cancer Center, 1275 York Avenue, New York, NY 10065, USA
* Corresponding author. UHN Breast Restoration Program, Division of Plastic and Reconstructive Surgery, Toronto General Hospital, North Building, 8N – 871, 200 Elizabeth Street, Toronto, Ontario M5G 2C4, Canada.
E-mail address: Toni.zhong@uhn.ca

outcomes research studies now cover a broad range of topics such as quality of care, process of care, access, decision making, prediction rules, and effectiveness. Although most people still equate outcomes research with observational epidemiologic study designs only, outcome studies today and in the future include randomized controlled trials (RCT). Furthermore, outcomes research uses a wide variety of analytical methods such as analysis of administrative databases, decision analysis, propensity scoring as a way of minimizing bias in observational studies, and the use of instrumental variables in access to care research. Also, in addition to the traditional primary outcomes such as disease status end points, outcomes research now assesses a broad range of end points such as health-related quality of life (Hr-QOL), patient satisfaction, and cost. **Fig. 1** shows a conceptualization of the relationship between study questions, research design, end points, and applications that define outcomes research that has been adapted from Lee and colleagues.[3]

CLINICAL TRIALS

Outcomes research serves to complement, rather than compete with, clinical trials, because it attempts to better understand how treatment in the real world affects a wide range of outcomes outside the controlled trial setting. Because Hr-QOL, patient satisfaction, and cost are usually considered end points for outcomes research, a classically designed phase III clinical trial would be under the umbrella term of clinical outcomes research when it uses 1 of these as its primary end point (see **Fig. 1**). Thus, outcomes research, regardless of its design methodology, is designed to approximate what health care is intended to achieve: improvements in functional status and Hr-QOL.[1] Thus, the intersection between outcomes research and clinical trials is a natural point of convergence in plastic surgery research in which the goal of treatment is to restore function and improve Hr-QOL.

In a review by McCarthy and colleagues,[4] who examined all level I evidence publications in 5 leading plastic surgery journals from 1978 to 2009, although the number of RCTs and meta-analyses were increasing, they were still limited in number. In addition, most of the studies did not appropriately use blinding, randomization, power analyses, or consider cost. Other investigators also independently found that well-design RCTs are uncommon in the plastic surgery literature,[5–7] likely because of the numerous challenges

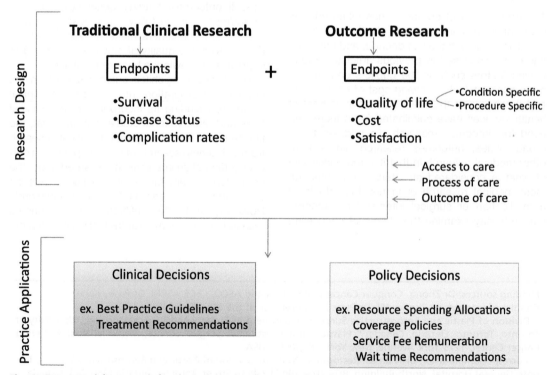

Fig. 1. Conceptual framework for the intersection between clinical research and outcomes research. (*Modified from* Lee SJ, Earle CC, Weeks JC. Outcomes research in oncology: history, conceptual framework, and trends in the literature. J Natl Cancer Inst 2000;92(3):195; with permission.)

associated with designing a surgical trial. First, it is often difficult to motivate surgeons to participate in a randomized surgical trial because most surgeons tend to have a preferred surgical technique and may not be willing to perform the experimental technique. Thus, the lack of clinical equipoise would preclude the recruitment of participating surgeons. Patient accrual may similarly be hindered if there are strong patient preferences or if the surgical intervention in question becomes too widespread. Second, blinding and concealment can be challenging because the surgeon can rarely be blinded to the procedure being performed, and it may also be impossible for the patient to be blinded to the treatment if the result is physically visible. Third, and perhaps the greatest impediment to conducting an RCT, are the required resources (monetary, physical, and human). As a result, RCTs often involve only a small number of academic centers with high volumes of patients and access to full-time dedicated study personnel.[8]

Well-conceived and executed clinical trials should be at the frontier of clinical outcomes research in plastic surgery. To achieve this goal, plastic surgeons, especially those in academic centers, must first resist the powerful temptation to prematurely draw anecdotally based conclusions and become more open to participating in surgical trials. Second, if blinding the surgeon or the patient is not ethical or feasible, then a blinded third-party assessor may be used to evaluate the outcome. Third, collective research efforts need to be fostered internationally to produce results that are adequately powered and can be generalized in the setting of multicenter trials as well as shared network research databases. Fourth, the future ability of plastic surgeons to conduct meaningful, high-quality clinical trials will rely heavily on plastic surgery foundations, academic associations, and research agencies to provide funding, mentoring, and capacity building in an area in which there is a gap in knowledge and expertise. Future improvement in the quality of RCTs in plastic surgery will result in more published studies in prestigious journals that will adhere to the standards for conducting and reporting of RCTs using the Consolidated Standards of Reporting Trials (CONSORT) statement.[9]

OBSERVATIONAL STUDIES

Although the RCT study design is often considered to be the epitome of clinical research, the only basic difference between an RCT and a well-conducted prospective observational study is the allocation of patients. In an RCT, the allocation is random; in an observation study, there is always the possibility of selection bias on the part of the provider or patient. In recent years, biostatisticians have promoted propensity scores as a method of reducing bias and improving the quality of results generated from observational studies.[10] Propensity scores provide a creative solution to dealing with the large number of confounding variables that are inherent in observational studies. In concept, a propensity score is found by using the confounding variables as predictors of the group to which a subject belongs, a step that is generally accomplished by using logistic regression. For example, in a cohort study, because the outcome is known for the subjects in the cohort, the confounding variables are used to develop a logistic regression equation to predict whether or not a patient has the outcome. This prediction, based on a combination of the confounding variables, is calculated for all subjects and then used as the confounding variable in subsequent analyses.[11] Proponents of this technique maintain that a propensity score is a superior approach to controlling for confounding variables, compared with multiple regressions or analysis of covariance, especially in analyzing large datasets. Because the area of health services research using epidemiologic or population-based data will continue to flourish in plastic surgery, sophisticated and novel methods of analysis, such as propensity score, will be more widely applied.

OUTCOME MEASURE DEVELOPMENT

In recent years, clinical researchers in plastic surgery have increasingly sought to improve understanding of the patient perspective on outcomes. This improvement has been facilitated by the development of a new generation of patient-reported outcome (PRO) instruments that can be used to reliably quantify subjective outcomes such as satisfaction and quality of life. In the past, most of the plastic surgery literature was populated with ad-hoc patient questionnaires that did not adhere to an acceptable level of validity or reliability. As a result, findings from such studies could only be interpreted with great caution. Other studies have relied on the use of generic PRO instruments, such as the Short Form 36. Although such instruments may be valid and reliable, they have low sensitivity to change and thus may fail to adequately measure the impact of plastic surgery procedures and changes in outcomes over time.

Newer generation, plastic surgery–specific PRO instruments such as the BREAST-Q and FACE-Q,[12–14] represent an important advancement in this area. Developed and validated according to rigorous international standards,[15,16] such condition-specific PRO instruments can provide clinically meaningful data to guide surgical advancements, patient selection, and clinical care. This emphasis on clinical meaning is a key attribute of new-generation PRO instruments. When developed using strong qualitative methodology in combination with modern psychometric analyses (Rasch), such instruments can offer valid, reliable, and meaningful quantification of the patient experience and perception of outcome.[17]

QUALITATIVE STUDY DESIGNS

Although quantitative methodology is important in outcomes research, it lacks the ability to provide a detailed insight into the patient's personal physical, psychological, and social experiences. In contrast, qualitative methodology is the ideal tool for exploring these complex domains and the interplay between them. Rather than being confined to the limits of a Likert scale or check boxes, patients are asked to express their feelings and thoughts, thus the ability to put their experiences into their own words is the central tenet of qualitative research.[18] Shauver and Chung[18] found in 2010 that there were only 11 published qualitative studies of plastic surgery topics at that time.[19] Although the number of qualitative studies in plastic surgery is still low, their importance is increasingly recognized, because there are now publications of qualitative studies on an array of patient experiences with conditions such as mastectomy defects, open tibial fractures, sacrectomies, and pectus excavacum.[20–23] In an era in which the quality of surgical care is under close scrutiny, and both public and private payers wish to steer surgical patients to high-quality providers (so-called value-based purchasing), qualitative methods will provide detailed insight to help surgeons better understand the needs and expectations of their patients.[24]

HEALTH SERVICES RESEARCH

The term health services research is defined as the integration of epidemiologic, sociologic, economic, and other analytical sciences in the study of health services. The aim of the research is evaluation, particularly in terms of structure, process, output, and outcome.[25] In plastic surgery, published studies in health services research have increased in number in the last 10 years. The most well-researched health service in plastic surgery is postmastectomy breast reconstruction (**Table 1**). These patterns of care studies

using large administrative databases and cancer registries have shown that patient factors such as increased age, nonwhite race, and low income; geographic factors such as living in the Midwest United States or a nonurban location; and cancer factors such as advanced breast cancer stage and anticipated need for radiation therapy all are associated with a lower rate of postmastectomy breast reconstruction.[26–41] Other population-based health services that have also been studied in plastic surgery have included craniofacial surgery, burns, breast augmentation, cosmetic surgery, hand and wrist surgery, and uncommon skin malignancies such as Merkel cell carcinoma and primary mucinous cancer of skin.[42–50] In light of the 2 dominant and opposing themes in the United States (the soaring cost of health care and the public perception that quality of care is substandard), future research directed at examining the relationships between need, supply, cost, and outcome of essential plastic surgery services through health services research will be in high demand.

COST AND EFFECTIVENESS RESEARCH

An economic analysis uses a set of quantitative methods to compare 2 or more interventions with respect to their resource use and expected outcomes.[51] Although there are various different types of economic evaluations, a cost-utility analysis integrates both cost and a health utility measure by weighting outcomes according to their perceived value. Health utilities are used to calculate quality-adjusted life-years (QALYs), which provide a value for the increase in quality and quantity of life as a result of a particular intervention. QALYs is the ideal outcome measure for an intervention when Hr-QOL is the most important outcome, thus it may be used to study most reconstructive surgeries. The incremental cost-utility ratio (ICUR) is the difference in QALYs gained between the 2 interventions, and provides a common metric by which a new technique can be compared with the standard technique.[42] Thus, in the current era of increased financial restraints and fiscal responsibility, QALY and ICUR are powerful tools to inform resource allocation decisions among groups in the population or the choice of treatment of patient groups.[51]

INTEGRATION OF OUTCOMES RESEARCH INTO GOVERNING BODIES

The outcomes research movement began as a response to the sociopolitical changes in our health care system a decade ago, and since then

Table 1
Summary of breast reconstruction population-based studies

Investigators	Year	Database	Rate of Utilization
Regional Canadian Population-based Databases			
Baxter et al,[26] 2005	1984/1985 1995/1996	Ontario (CIHI)	Overall rate 7.9% 1984/1985 Overall rate 7.7% 1994/1994
Barnsley et al,[25] 2008	1991/2001	Nova Scotia Medical Services Insurance and CIHI	Overall average rate 3.8% for 10 y 23% IBR 74% DBR
United States Nationwide Population-based Databases			
Polednak,[33] 2000	1988–1995	SEER registries	Overall 8.1% 1988: 4.3% 1995: 10.8%
Alderman et al,[27] 2003	1998	SEER registries	15%
Alderman et al,[28] 2006	1998–2002	SEER registries	16.5%
United States Regional Population Based			
Polednak,[32] 2001	1992–1997	Connecticut Tumor Registry (part of SEER) and Connecticut's Hospital Discharge Database	Average rate of 12.5% Rate increased with each year, highest in 1996: 15.6%
Polednak,[31] 1999	1988–1995	Connecticut Tumor Registry (part of SEER)	1988: 9.1% 1995: 8.5%
Tseng et al,[37] 2010	2000–2006	Greater Sacramento SEER	20.2% +
United States Nationwide Hospital Based			
Morrow et al,[24] 2001	1985–1990 and 1994–1995	NCDB	1985–1990: 3.4% 1994–1995: 8.3%
Christian et al,[29] 2006	1997–2002	8 NCCN centers	Overall rate of 42% 95% were IBR
Reuben et al,[34] 2009	1998–2003	Nationwide inpatient sample	23.6%
United States Regional Institution Hospital Based			
Desch et al,[30] 1999	1989–1991	Virginia Cancer Registry linked to Blue Cross and Blue Shield	1989–1991: 16%
Rosson et al,[35] 2008	1995–2004	Maryland Hospital Discharge Database	27.9%

Abbreviations: CIHI, Canadian Institute for Health Information; DBR, delayed breast reconstruction; EBR, early breast reconstruction; IBR, immediate breast reconstruction; NCCN, National Comprehensive Cancer Network; NCDB, National Cancer Database; SEER, Surveillance, End Results and Epidemiology.

it has entered into many key aspects of clinical research. Developing at the same time as outcomes research is the growth in health services research/governing bodies whose responsibility is to ensure the quality of patient care, promote physician-patient relationships, and provide credible information to assist third-party payers in determining reimbursement policies.[3] In oncology, the American Society of Clinical Oncology has a health services research group whose primary function is the development of practice guidelines, conduct of technology assessment, and the development of standardized parameters and definitions to use in outcomes research.[52] We anticipate that a similar research/governing body will be formed within the American Society of Plastic Surgeons in the foreseeable future.

SUMMARY

This article informs readers of the key areas in outcomes research that have experienced the most rapid growth in plastic surgery and that will continue to dominate in the future. Higher quality RCTs with multicenter collaboration that adhere to the CONSORT framework will generate more valid findings that can also be generalized. Traditional observational studies that use more novel and sophisticated analytical tools such as propensity score will decrease bias and improve the quality of nonexperimental studies. Studies that integrate both quantitative methods using validated conditions and procedure-specific PRO instruments as well as the qualitative method will provide insight into important patient-centered issues such as expectation and satisfaction. In addition, both health services research and cost-effectiveness research will likely thrive in the future as difficult questions about the quality and the cost of surgical care to the society are increasingly posed by policy makers, third-party payers, hospitals, and patients.

REFERENCES

1. Kane RL. Understanding health care outcomes research. 2nd edition. Sudbury (MA): Jones and Bartlett Publishers; 2006.
2. Jefford M, Stockler MR, Tattersall MH. Outcomes research: what is it and why does it matter? Intern Med J 2003;33:110–8.
3. Lee SJ, Earle CC, Weeks JC. Outcomes research in oncology: history, conceptual framework, and trends in the literature. J Natl Cancer Inst 2000;92(3):195.
4. McCarthy JE, Chatterjee A, McKelvey TG, et al. A detailed analysis of level I evidence (randomized controlled trials and meta-analyses) in five plastic surgery journals to date: 1978 to 2009. Plast Reconstr Surg 2010;126(5):1774–8.
5. Offer GJ, Perks AG. In search of evidence-based plastic surgery: the problems faced by the specialty. Br J Plast Surg 2000;53(5):427–33.
6. Karri V. Randomised clinical trials in plastic surgery: survey of output and quality of reporting. J Plast Reconstr Aesthet Surg 2006;59:787.
7. Veiga Filho J, Castro AA, Veiga DF, et al. Quality of reports of randomized clinical trials in plastic surgery. Plast Reconstr Surg 2005;115(1):320–3.
8. McCarthy CM. Randomized controlled trials. Plast Reconstr Surg 2011;127(4):1707–12.
9. Begg C, Cho M, Eastwood S, et al. Improving the quality of reporting of randomized controlled trials: the CONSORT statement. JAMA 1996;276:637–9.
10. D'Agostino RH Jr. Propensity score methods for bias reduction in the comparison of a treatment to non-randomized control group. Stat Med 1998;17:2265–81.
11. Rubin DB. Estimating causal effects from large data sets using propensity scores. Ann Intern Med 1997;127:757–63.
12. Pusic AL, Klassen AF, Scott AM, et al. Development of a new patient-reported outcome measure for breast surgery: the BREAST-Q. Plast Reconstr Surg 2009;124(2):345–53.
13. Cano SJ, Klassen AF, Scott AM, et al. The BREAST-Q: further validation in independent clinical samples. Plast Reconstr Surg 2012;129(2):293–302.
14. Klassen AF, Cano SJ, Scott A, et al. Measuring patient-reported outcomes in facial aesthetic patients: development of the FACE-Q. Facial Plast Surg 2010;26(4):303–9.
15. Scientific Advisory Committee of the Medical Outcomes Trust. Assessing health status and quality of life instruments: attributes and review criteria. Qual Life Res 2002;11:193.
16. Food and Drug Administration. Patient reported outcome measures: use in medical product development to support labeling claims. 2006. Available at: www.fda.gov/cber/gdlns/prolbl.pdf. Accessed August 30, 2012.
17. Zhong T, McCarthy C, Min S, et al. Patient satisfaction and health-related quality of life after autologous tissue breast reconstruction: a prospective analysis of early postoperative outcomes. Cancer 2012;118(6):1701–9. http://dx.doi.org/10.1002/cncr.26417.
18. Shauver MJ, Chung KC. A guide to qualitative research in plastic surgery. Plast Reconstr Surg 2010;126(3):1089–97.
19. Shauver MS, Aravind MS, Chung KC. A qualitative study of recovery from type III-B and III-C tibial fractures. Ann Plast Surg 2011;66(1):73–9.
20. Davidge KM, Eskicioglu C, Lipa J, et al. Qualitative assessment of patient experiences following sacrectomy. J Surg Oncol 2010;101(6):447–50.
21. Snell L, McCarthy C, Klassen A, et al. Clarifying the expectations of patients undergoing implant breast reconstruction: a qualitative study. Plast Reconstr Surg 2010;126(6):1825–30.
22. Galvin R, Milstein A. Large employers' new strategies in health care. N Engl J Med 2002;347(12):939–42.
23. National Library of Medicine. Medical subject headings. Available at: http://www.nlm.nij.gov/mesh. Accessed August 30, 2012.
24. Morrow M, Scott SK, Menck HR, et al. Factors influencing the use of breast reconstruction postmastectomy: a National Cancer Database study. J Am Coll Surg 2001;192(1):1–8.
25. Barnsley GP, Sigurdson L, Kirkland S. Barriers to breast reconstruction after mastectomy in Nova Scotia. Can J Surg 2008;51(6):447–52.
26. Baxter N, Goel V, Semple JL. Utilization and regional variation of breast reconstruction in Canada. Plast Reconstr Surg 2005;115:338–9.
27. Alderman AK, McMahon L Jr, Wilkins EG. The national utilization of immediate and early delayed breast reconstruction and the effect of sociodemographic factors. Plast Reconstr Surg 2003;111(2):695–703.

28. Alderman AK, Wei Y, Birkmeyer JD. Use of breast reconstruction after mastectomy following the Women's Health and Cancer Rights Act. JAMA 2006;295:387–8.

29. Christian CK, Niland J, Edge SB, et al. A multi-institutional analysis of the socioeconomic determinants of breast reconstruction. Ann Surg 2006;243:241–9.

30. Desch CE, Penberthy LT, Hillner BE, et al. A sociodemographic and economic comparison of breast reconstruction, mastectomy, and conservative surgery. Surgery 1999;125:441–7.

31. Polednak AP. Postmastectomy breast reconstruction in Connecticut: trends and predictors. Plast Reconstr Surg 1999;104(3):669–73.

32. Polednak AP. How frequent is postmastectomy breast reconstructive surgery? A study linking two statewide databases. Plast Reconstr Surg 2001; 108(1):73–7.

33. Polednak AP. Geographic variation in postmastectomy breast reconstruction rates. Plast Reconstr Surg 2000;106(2):298–301.

34. Reuben BC, Manwaring J, Neumayer LA. Recent trends and predictors in immediate breast reconstruction after mastectomy in the United States. Am J Surg 2009;198(2):237–43.

35. Rosson GD, Singh NK, Ahuja N, et al. Multilevel analysis of the impact of community vs patient factors on access to immediate breast reconstruction following mastectomy in Maryland. Arch Surg 2008;143(11):1076–81.

36. Tseng JF, Kronowitz SJ, Sun CC, et al. The effect of ethnicity on immediate reconstruction rates after mastectomy for breast cancer. Cancer 2004; 101(7):1514–23.

37. Tseng WH, Stevenson TR, Canter RJ, et al. Sacramento area breast cancer epidemiology study: use of postmastectomy breast reconstruction along the rural-to-urban continuum. Plast Reconstr Surg 2010;126:1815–24.

38. Joslyn SA. Patterns of care for immediate and early delayed breast reconstruction following mastectomy. Plast Reconstr Surg 2005;115(5):1289–96.

39. Kruper L, Holt A, Xu XX, et al. Disparities in reconstruction rates after mastectomy: patterns of care and factors associated with the use of breast reconstruction in southern California. Ann Surg Oncol 2011;18:2158–65.

40. Thoma A, Ignacy TA. Health services research: impact of quality of life instruments on craniofacial surgery. J Craniofac Surg 2012;23(1):283–7.

41. De Putter CE, Selles RW, Polinder S, et al. Economic impact of hand and wrist injuries: health-care costs and productivity costs in a population-based study. J Bone Joint Surg Am 2012;94(9):e56.

42. Albornoz CR, Bach PB, Pusic AL, et al. The influence of sociodemographic factors and hospital characteristics on the method of breast reconstruction, including microsurgery: a U.S. population-based study. Plast Reconstr Surg 2012;129(5):1071–9.

43. Haik J, Grabov-Nardini G, Goldan O, et al. Expanded reverse abdominoplasty for reconstruction of burns in the epigastric region and the inframammary fold in female patients. J Burn Care Res 2007;28(6):849–53.

44. Chung KC, Shauver MJ, Yin H, et al. Variations in the use of internal fixation for distal radial fracture in the United States Medicare population. J Bone Joint Surg Am 2011;93(23):2154–62.

45. Kukko H, Böhling T, Koljonen V, et al. Merkel cell carcinoma - a population-based epidemiological study in Finland with a clinical series of 181 cases. Eur J Cancer 2012;48(5):737–42.

46. Javo IM, Sørlie T. Psychosocial predictors of an interest in cosmetic surgery among young Norwegian women: a population-based study. Plast Reconstr Surg 2010;126(2):687–8 [author reply: 688].

47. Javo IM, Sørlie T. Psychosocial predictors of an interest in cosmetic surgery among young Norwegian women: a population-based study. Plast Reconstr Surg 2009;124(6):2142–8.

48. Hvilsom GB, Hölmich LR, Henriksen TF, et al. Local complications after cosmetic breast augmentation: results from the Danish Registry for Plastic Surgery of the Breast. Plast Reconstr Surg 2009;124(3): 919–25.

49. Thoma A, McKnight LL. Quality-adjusted life-year as a surgical outcome measure: a primer for plastic surgeons. Plast Reconstr Surg 2010;125(4):1279–87.

50. American Society of Clinical Oncology. Committee: Health Services Research. Available at: http://asco.infostreet.com/prof. Accessed August 30, 2012.

51. Forrest CB, Shipman SA, Dougherty D, et al. Outcomes research in pediatric settings: recent trends and future directions. Pediatrics 2003; 111(1):171.

52. Moher D, Schulz KF, Altman D, CONSORT Group (Consolidated Standards of Reporting Trials). The CONSORT statement: revised recommendations for improving the quality of reports of parallel-group randomized trials. JAMA 2001;285(15):1987–91.

Index

Note: Page numbers of article titles are in **boldface** type.

Clin Plastic Surg 40 (2013) 359–361
http://dx.doi.org/10.1016/S0094-1298(13)00010-2
0094-1298/13/$ – see front matter © 2013 Elsevier Inc. All rights reserved.

Moving?

Make sure your subscription moves with you!

To notify us of your new address, find your **Clinics Account Number** (located on your mailing label above your name), and contact customer service at:

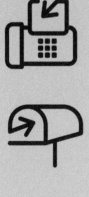

Email: journalscustomerservice-usa@elsevier.com

800-654-2452 (subscribers in the U.S. & Canada)
314-447-8871 (subscribers outside of the U.S. & Canada)

Fax number: 314-447-8029

Elsevier Health Sciences Division
Subscription Customer Service
3251 Riverport Lane
Maryland Heights, MO 63043

*To ensure uninterrupted delivery of your subscription, please notify us at least 4 weeks in advance of move.

Moving?

Make sure your subscription moves with you!

To notify us of your new address, find your Clinics Account number (located on your mailing label above your name), and contact customer service at:

Email: journalscustomerservice-usa@elsevier.com

800-654-2452 (subscribers in the U.S. & Canada)
314-447-8871 (subscribers outside of the U.S. & Canada)

Fax number: 314-447-8029

Elsevier Health Sciences Division
Subscription Customer Service
3251 Riverport Lane
Maryland Heights, MO 63043

Printed and bound by CPI Group (UK) Ltd, Croydon, CR0 4YY

03/10/2024

01040346-0008